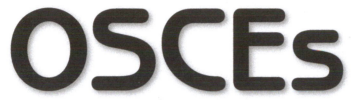

The Easy Guide to

Focused History Taking for

OSCEs

Second Edition

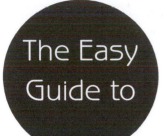

The Easy Guide to

Focused History Taking for

OSCEs

Second Edition

David McCollum MB ChB

GP Registrar, Leeds

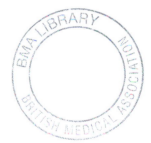

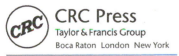

CRC Press
Taylor & Francis Group
Boca Raton London New York

CRC Press is an imprint of the
Taylor & Francis Group, an **informa** business

CRC Press
Taylor & Francis Group
6000 Broken Sound Parkway NW, Suite 300
Boca Raton, FL 33487-2742

© 2017 by Taylor & Francis Group, LLC
CRC Press is an imprint of Taylor & Francis Group, an Informa business

No claim to original U.S. Government works

Printed in Great Britain by Ashford Colour Press Ltd

International Standard Book Number-13: 978-1-138-19652-0 (Paperback)
International Standard Book Number-13: 978-1-138-74328-1 (Hardback)

Library of Congress Cataloging-in-Publication Data

Names: McCollum, David (Doctor), author.
Title: The easy guide to focused history taking for OSCEs / David McCollum.
Other titles: Focused history taking for OSCEs | Easy guide to focused
history taking for objective structured clinical examinations
Description: Second edition. | Boca Raton : CRC Press, [2017] | Preceded by
Focused history taking for OSCEs : a comprehensive guide for medical
students / David McCollum [and others]. c2013. | Includes index.
Identifiers: LCCN 2016054173| ISBN 9781138196520 (paperback : alk. paper) |
ISBN 9781138743281 (hardback : alk. paper) | ISBN 9781315181783 (master eBook) |
Subjects: | MESH: Medical History Taking--methods | Physical Examination |
Examination Questions
Classification: LCC R834.5 | NLM WB 18.2 | DDC 610.76--dc23
LC record available at https://lccn.loc.gov/2016054173

Visit the Taylor & Francis Web site at
http://www.taylorandfrancis.com

and the CRC Press Web site at
http://www.crcpress.com

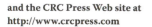

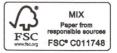

Contents

Contents

Foreword to the first edition

The OSCE examination or its equivalent is rapidly becoming the gold standard in how the clinical knowledge, acumen and skills of undergraduate medical students and postgraduate medical trainees are tested in a controlled and reproducible clinicomimetic environment.

In Manchester at any one time we have in excess of 2200 medical students. Our programme is specifically designed to train students to be independent learners and to set them up for life as doctors in the rapidly changing world of modern medicine and healthcare.

For a student, this book is a perfect learning resource for approaching a whole series of clinical problems. But it goes further, eloquently showing how to construct a successful approach to any clinical problem. I thoroughly recommend this book to all clinical students. If you read it you will learn a great deal about specific medical problems, see how to approach common clinical scenarios and, perhaps more importantly, learn how to analyse a clinical setting and efficiently extract the information necessary for diagnosis and the initiation of management.

This really is a super little book that goes further than just showing how to pass an exam, but rather equips the reader with a philosophical approach to any clinical problem. Congratulations to all the authors, but especially David McCollum, who as a fifth-year medical student at Manchester was the life force behind this book.

Professor Anthony Freemont
Head of Undergraduate Medical Education
and
Professor of Osteoarticular Pathology
University of Manchester

Foreword to the second edition

As a GP trainer and training programme director on the Leeds GP training scheme, I spend a lot of time teaching consultation skills. It was a real pleasure to read this book and see the emphasis on consultation and communication skills, starting with the excellent Calgary–Cambridge model. Fully exploring the patients' perspective of their illness (including their ideas, concerns and expectations) is not only polite and courteous but also an easy and powerful way of collecting important and relevant information about the case.

All of the cases in this book can present in a 10-minute GP appointment, and it is our communication skills every bit as much as our other medical skills that enable us to formulate a management plan. General practice is a highly rewarding career where these communication skills are fundamental to daily practice.

I heartily recommend this book, particularly the introductory chapter, which highlights how you can construct a medical interview in a time-efficient and effective manner. Good luck with your exams.

Dr Simon O'Hara
General Practitioner
Training Programme Director
Leeds VTS

Preface

A good general practitioner will tell you that most diagnoses are made from clinical history alone and not from examinations or investigations. Following on from the success of the first edition, *Focused History Taking for OSCEs*, comes the second edition, *The Easy Guide to Focused History Taking for OSCEs*.

The second edition incorporates feedback received from the first edition and ensures the text is up-to-date at the time of publishing. The introductory chapter tackles how to construct histories using the Calgary–Cambridge framework and how to approach history-based OSCE stations. This includes tips from recently qualified doctors and a highly respected examiner. New features for this edition include blue boxes within each history to highlight the red flag symptoms, references to current NICE clinical knowledge summaries and guidelines, as well as more illustrations. Whilst maintaining a simple layout, the histories have been re-structured to mirror the Calgary–Cambridge model of consultations that is widely taught throughout the United Kingdom and abroad. New and updated histories have been written for this edition with each history also considering differential diagnoses, investigations and management.

This book is a comprehensive guide to history taking to suit modern medical student examination purposes. This book provides a database of histories based on common scenarios in student examinations across the United Kingdom.

David McCollum
GP Registrar
Leeds

Acknowledgements

Colleagues from many specialities throughout medicine and surgery have contributed to the production of this book. Each chapter has been written by well-respected doctors and reviewed by experts in their respective field. I would like to thank those, including several family members, who have helped either in writing or reviewing chapters in this book as well as the previous edition.

AUTHORS FROM THE FIRST EDITION

Professor Peter McCollum, MB BCh MA MCh FRCSI FRCSEd, Professor of Vascular Surgery/Hon Consultant Vascular Surgeon, Hull York Medical School/Hull & East Yorkshire Hospitals NHS Trust. As co-author of the first edition, Peter helped to write the introductory and surgical chapters in the first edition of the book as well as reviewing the other chapters in the book. Peter has extensive experience in examining at all levels of medical and surgical training including medical student OSCEs across the United Kingdom. He has been a member of council and deputy exam convenor in the Royal College of Surgeons of Edinburgh.

Dr Graham McCollum, MB BS BSc, Ophthalmology registrar and co-author of the first edition. Graham helped to write the general medicine, cardiorespiratory, urology and ophthalmology chapters in the first edition. Graham graduated from Hull/York Medical School in July 2012.

Dr Priha McCollum, MB ChB, GP registrar and co-author of the first edition. Priha helped to write the gastroenterology and obstetrics and gynaecology chapters, as well as reviewing the other chapters in the book. Priha graduated from the University of Manchester in July 2011.

CONTRIBUTORS TO THE FIRST EDITION

Dr Thomas Hansen (Acute Care Common Stem trainee) and Mr Kevin Morris (Consultant Neurosurgeon) for helping to write and review the neurology chapter, respectively; Dr Suparna Dasgupta (Consultant Paediatrician) for helping to review the paediatric chapter; Dr Amit Sindhi (Specialist Registrar, Psychiatry) for helping to write and review the psychiatry chapter; Mr Sachchidananda Maiti and Mrs Wendy Noble (Consultants, Obstetrics & Gynaecology) for helping to review the obstetrics and gynaecology chapter; Dr Rachel Gorodkin (Consultant Rheumatologist) for helping to review the musculoskeletal and general medicine chapters; Dr Patrick Newman (General Practitioner) for helping to review the general medicine chapter; Dr David Ahearn (Consultant, Elderly Medicine) for reviewing the gastroenterology chapter; Professor Andrew Clark (Professor of Cardiology) and

Dr Simon Hart (Consultant Respiratory Physician) for helping to review the cardiorespiratory chapter; Mr Sigurd Kraus (Consultant Urologist) for helping to review the urology chapter; Mr Jim Innes (Consultant Ophthalmologist) for helping to review the ophthalmology chapter.

CONTRIBUTORS TO THE SECOND EDITION

Dr Sharfaraz Salam (Neurology Clinical Fellow) and Mr Justin Murphy (Consultant Head and Neck Surgeon) for reviewing the neurology and ENT sections, respectively.

Author

David McCollum, MB ChB, graduated from the University of Manchester's Medical School in July 2012 with MB ChB. He completed his foundation training at University Hospital of South Manchester and The Christie Hospital in Manchester. His foundation jobs included general surgery, general medicine, respiratory medicine, emergency medicine, general practice and oncology at the renowned Christie Hospital. He now lives and works in Leeds and is in the final year of the Leeds GP Vocational Training Scheme. As part of this training, he has done jobs in elderly medicine, emergency medicine and ENT, as well as having worked as a GP registrar at Leeds Student Medical Practice and in his current job at Meanwood Health Practice.

David McCollum's interests include medical education, rheumatology and ENT, for which he is looking to pursue additional qualifications. He has previously been involved in co-ordinating regional teaching events in Manchester in the past, including *Fit For Finals,* a revision course designed for final year medical students. He is keen to become more involved in undergraduate and postgraduate education after gaining his completion of training certificate in general practice.

Abbreviations

A&E	Accident and Emergency department		FH	Family history
ABG	Arterial blood gas		FSH	Follicle-stimulating hormone
ACE	Angiotensin-converting enzyme		G6PD	Glucose-6-phosphatase dehydrogenase
ACS	Acute coronary syndrome		GIT	Gastro-intestinal tract
ADHD	Attention-deficit hyperactivity disorder		GORD	Gastro-oesophageal reflux disease
ALP	Alkaline phosphatase		GUM	Genito-urinary medicine
ALS	Advanced life support		GUT	Genito-urinary tract
ALT	Alanine transaminase		GP	General practitioner
ANA	Anti-nuclear antibodies		GT	Glutamyl transferase
ANCA	Anti-neutrophil cytoplasmic antibodies		GTN	Gliceryl trinitrate
BMI	Body mass index		hCG	Human chorionic gonadotropin
BNP	Brain natriuretic peptide		HDL	High-density lipoprotein
BPH	Benign prostatic hyperplasia		HLA	Human leucocyte antigen
BPPV	Benign paroxysmal positional vertigo		HPC	History of presenting complaint
CBT	Cognitive behavioural therapy		HIV	Human immunodeficiency virus
CKS	Clinical knowledge summary		HPV	Human papilloma virus
CMV	Cytomegalovirus		HRT	Hormone replacement therapy
COCP	Combined oral contraceptive pill		IBD	Inflammatory bowel disease
COPD	Chronic obstructive pulmonary disorder		IDS	Irritable bowel syndrome
CRP	C-reactive protein		ICE	Ideas, concerns and expectations
CT	Computed tomography		ICP	Intracranial pressure
CTD	Connective tissue disorder		IHD	Ischaemic heart disease
CTPA	Computed tomography pulmonary angiography		IM	Intramuscular
			IMB	Intermenstrual bleeding
CVS	Cardiovascular system		IV	Intravenous
DAT	Dopamine transporter		KUB	Kidneys, ureter and bladder
DEXA	Dual-energy x-ray absorptiometry		LDL	Low-density lipoprotein
DH	Drug history		LFT	Liver function test
DMARD	Disease modifying anti-rheumatic drug		LH	Luteinising hormone
DVLA	Driver and vehicle licensing agency		LMN	Lower motor neuron
DVT	Deep vein thrombosis		LMP	Last menstrual period
EBV	Epstein-Barr virus		LOC	Loss of consciousness
ECG	Electrocardiography		LRTI	Lower respiratory tract infection
EEG	Electroencephalography		MDT	Multi-disciplinary team
eGFR	Estimated glomerular filtration rate		MRI	Magnetic resonance imaging
ENT	Ear, nose and throat		MSK	Musculoskeletal system
ESR	Erythrocyte sedimentation rate		MSU	Mid-stream urine sample
FAST	Focussed assessment with sonography for trauma		NAI	Non-accidental injury
			NS	Neurological system
FBC	Full blood count		NSAID	Non-steroidal anti-inflammatory drug

OSCE	Objective structured clinical examination
OSLER	Objective structured long examination record
PC	Presenting complaint
PCB	Postcoital bleeding
PCI	Percutaneous coronary intervention
PCR	Polymerase chain reaction
PE	Pulmonary embolism
PET	Positron emission tomography
PMB	Postmenopausal bleeding
PMH	Past medical history
PR	Per-rectal
PRN	Pro re nata (as required)
PSA	Prostate-specific antigen
PUO	Pyrexia of unknown origin
PUVA	Psoralen Ultraviolet A (photochemotherapy)
PV	Per-vaginal
RA	Rheumatoid arthritis
RS	Respiratory system

SH	Social history
SIADH	Syndrome of inappropriate antidiuretic hormone hypersecretion
SLE	Systemic lupus erythematosus
SP	Simulated patient
SSRI	Selective serotonin re-uptake inhibitor
STI	Sexually transmitted infection
TB	Tuberculosis
TFT	Thyroid function test
TNF	Tumour necrosis factor
U&E	Urea and electrolyte
UMN	Upper motor neuron
URTI	Upper respiratory tract infection
USS	Ultrasound scan
UTI	Urinary tract infection
VEGF	Vascular endothelial growth factor
y/o	Years old

Taking a focused history in OSCEs – The Calgary–Cambridge model

An OSCE history station is quite similar to the real life situation faced by general practitioners where they often have only 5–10 minutes to take a history (± examining the patient) and generate a working diagnosis with a management plan. As such, the Calgary–Cambridge model of interview is extremely useful in its application.

One of the challenges medical students and doctors alike often face is the perceived battle between the traditional medical history and the modern communication model of interview. The communication model however should be viewed as the *process* of interview and the traditional medical history viewed as the content you wish to obtain. Using communication models such as the Calgary–Cambridge model allows you to acquire more information in the history, including sequencing of events and the patient's perspective of the illness. The process allows collection of past medical history, drug history, etc., in the background information aspect of the model.

The Calgary–Cambridge model is the most commonly used and promoted model in medical schools throughout the United Kingdom and abroad. The core concepts of the model are summarised in the following sections.

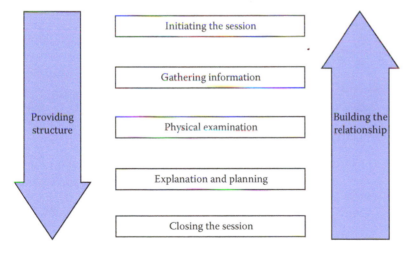

The Calgary–Cambridge model of consultation (Kurtz and Silverman).

INITIATING THE SESSION

PREPARATION

- **Before starting** – ensure appropriate positioning of seats and the absence of physical barriers between patient and doctor; paper/computer to document if required.

ESTABLISH INITIAL RAPPORT

- **Greeting** – greet the patient, confirm his/her name and date of birth.
- **Introduction** – introduce yourself and describe your role; explain the reason for interview, obtain consent and explain confidentiality if necessary (*as a doctor, this is generally assumed; as a medical student, however, it is polite to explain if the interview is for your own benefit, discuss confidentiality and seek their consent in this instance*).
- **Respect** – demonstrate interest, concern and respect for the patient as a person; ensure the patient's comfort.

IDENTIFY THE REASON(S) FOR CONSULTATION

- **Opening question** – use an appropriate opening question to identify problems/issues that the patient wishes to discuss (e.g. "What concerns brought you to the hospital/clinic?").
- **Listen** – listen attentively without interrupting the patient's opening statement.
- **Screening** – check and confirm the list of problems or issues that the patient wishes to cover ("What other problems have you noticed?" or "Is there anything else you would like to bring to my attention?").
- **Agenda** – negotiate an agenda taking both the patient's and physician's needs into account; in most OSCEs this will be self-evident to both parties.

GATHERING INFORMATION

BIOMEDICAL PERSPECTIVE

- **Sequence of events** – encourage the patients to tell their story from the beginning.
- **Question style** – use both open-ended and closed questions; move appropriately from open to closed; at the start of the history use open questions predominantly, but as the history progresses more closed questions are often required to clarify finer details.
- **Listening** – listen attentively; allow the patient to complete statements without interruption; leave pauses for the patient to think before answering.
- **Facilitative response** – facilitate the patient's responses verbally and non-verbally (use encouragement, silence, repetition, paraphrasing, interpretation).
- **Cues** – pick up verbal and non-verbal cues (body language, speech, facial expression, affect); check them out and acknowledge as appropriate (e.g. "you seem tired"); look for props (medications, cigarette packets, Internet print-out etc.).

- **Clarification** – clarify any statements which are vague (e.g. "Could you explain what you mean by light headed?").
- **Time framing** – clarify dates and sequence of events.
- **Summarise** – periodically recap to verify your understanding and check chronology of events; allow the patient an opportunity to correct your interpretation and provide further information; this is particularly important in exams as it also allows the examiner to see that you have picked up and acknowledged important information.
- **Language** – use concise, clear and easily understood questions; avoid jargon.

> The biomedical perspective is the part of the process where the majority of the traditional "history of presenting complaint" is likely to be ascertained.

THE PATIENT'S PERSPECTIVE

- **Effects on life** – determine the effects of the problem(s) on the patient's life. Use cues previously mentioned by the patient to reflect on potential problems they might have.
- **Feelings and thoughts** – encourage the expression of the patient's feelings and thoughts; consider if the problem has had a significant effect on the patient's mood.
- **Ideas and concerns** – *fully* explore the patient's ideas (i.e. beliefs about what is causing their problems) and concerns regarding each problem (i.e. what are they concerned could be causing their problem *and* what in general is worrying them about their problem (e.g. no one to feed pets if admitted); establish their main concern; in an exam setting, a lot of key information may be locked behind fully exploring the patient's ideas and concerns (listen attentively for cues dropped along the way).
- **Expectations** – establish what the patient expects from the consultation.

BACKGROUND INFORMATION

- **Past medical history**
- **Drug and allergy history**
- **Family history**
- **Personal and social history** – much of this section can be picked up in the "patient's perspective" part of the history. This part of the history can therefore be a useful way of double-checking the effect the problem has had on their life. Consider their relationships, work-life and support mechanisms if relevant. Clearly this will be more important in certain histories e.g. of chronic disease than in others.
- **Systems review** – start with an open question e.g. "Have you noticed any other symptoms?" Then ask questions relevant to the appropriate system being explored as well as a quick check on other systems (only if relevant to the presenting problem).

PROVIDING STRUCTURE

- **Summarise** – at the end of a specific line of enquiry to confirm understanding before moving on to the next section.
- **Signpost** – when moving on to the next section use transitional statements to make it clear to the examiner that you have a logical sequence in your process.
- **Timing** – ensure you keep to time (in both an exam setting and reality, time is your most precious resource so make sure you use it as efficiently as possible).

BUILDING A RELATIONSHIP

NON-VERBAL BEHAVIOUR

- **To patient** – demonstrate an appropriate affect (e.g. eye contact, posture and position, movement, facial expression, use of voice).
- **Documentation** – if writing notes or using a computer, do so in a way that doesn't cause a barrier towards dialogue and rapport.

RAPPORT

- **Acknowledge** – accept legitimacy of the patient's views without being judgemental.
- **Empathy** – use empathy to communicate understanding of the patient's feelings.
- **Support** – express concern and a willingness to help along with appropriate self-care mechanisms.
- **Sensitivity** – deal sensitively with embarrassing topics; this is a closely scrutinised area in final year OSCEs due to the challenging nature of communication in such settings.

PATIENT INVOLVEMENT

- **Share thinking** – encourage patient involvement.
- **Explain rationale** – when asking sensitive questions, explain why this information is important for you to understand.

EXPLANATION AND PLANNING (OFTEN COMES UNDER "INFORMATION GIVING" IN AN OSCE FORMAT)

PROVIDE THE CORRECT AMOUNT AND TYPE OF INFORMATION

- **Assess the patient's starting point** – establish the patient's current understanding of their problem (if any) at the outset; establish how much the patient wants to know; remember even the brightest of patients only remembers so much.
- **Chunks and checks** – give information in digestible chunks; check for understanding; use the patient's response as a guide as to how much more is required.

- **Give explanations at the appropriate time** – avoid giving advice, information or reassurance prematurely (e.g. before important investigations are back to guide further discussions).

AID ACCURATE RECALL AND UNDERSTANDING

- **Organise explanation** – have a logical approach (e.g. discussing patient's symptoms → condition → possible investigations → shared management → addressing further concerns → follow-up).
- **Use explicit categorisation or signposting** – e.g. "There are three important things that I would like to discuss with you" (try to make the most important issue the first one); signpost to help the patient remember explanations.
- **Use repetition and summarise** – to reinforce and embed information in patients.
- **Use visual aids** – diagrams, models, written information and instructions.
- **Use simple language** – use concise, easily understood statements, avoid jargon; provide examples.
- **Check the patient's understanding** – e.g. by asking the patient to restate information in their own words; clarify if necessary.

ACHIEVE A SHARED UNDERSTANDING: INCORPORATE THE PATIENT'S ILLNESS FRAMEWORK

- **Relate explanations to the patient's perspective** – relate information to previously expressed ideas, concerns and expectations.
- **Provide opportunities and encourage the patient to contribute** – by asking questions, seeking clarification or expressing doubts; respond appropriately.
- **Identify and respond to verbal and non-verbal cues** – listen to the patient's responses to information; only give as much information as the patient wishes to take in at that consultation.
- **Elicit and assess the patient's reactions and feelings** – regarding information given, terms used; acknowledge and clarify where necessary; check whether they wish you to continue or discuss other concerns.

PLANNING: SHARED DECISION-MAKING

- **Share own thoughts** – ideas, thought processes and dilemmas.
- **Involve the patient** – offer suggestions rather than directives; "What would you like?"
- **Encourage patient contribution** – regarding their ideas, suggestions and preferences.
- **Negotiate** – negotiate a mutually acceptable plan.
- **Offer choice** – where desired, ask the patient to make informed choices and decisions.
- **Check with the patient** – if concerns have been addressed and whether they are happy with the negotiated plan.

CLOSING THE SESSION

- **End summary** – summarise the session briefly and clarify the plan of care.
- **Contract** – agree with the patient on the next steps for both patient and physician.

- **Safety net** – explain possible unexpected outcomes, when and how to seek help.
- **Final check** – check whether patient agrees and is comfortable with the plan and ask for any corrections, questions or other items to discuss.

The successful OSCE candidate is one who can successfully implement the Calgary–Cambridge model whilst ensuring that key elements of the history are not left out.

It is important to remember that patients in reality can be unreliable, and so internal cross-checking of event dates, past medical problems, etc., is a useful discipline. A simple example of this is hypertension, which will not be admitted by many patients simply because they consider that they no longer have it as they are now on anti-hypertensive medication. Use medications as a way of cross-checking the patient's past medical history. Thus, levothyroxine in the list of medications would indicate that the patient has hypothyroidism, even if not originally volunteered.

There is an understandable danger of becoming too mechanical while information gathering. Students need to do more than just "go through the motions" during the OSCE. A flat affect with little empathy comes across clearly to examiners and will not help the cause. Although it can be difficult to reconcile some scenarios with a clinical problem (e.g. a clearly normal simulated patient giving a history of jaundice), every effort should be made to consider the scenario in a real life concept.

A good general practitioner will tell you that most diagnoses are made from clinical history alone and not from examinations or investigations. For the purposes of this book, examination has intentionally been left out as this is well covered in other textbooks. In some OSCE scenarios, history and examination go alongside one another. However, it remains the case that a well-taken history will guide the candidate to a focussed and relevant examination.

In some stations, the emphasis will also be on information giving. It is important here to provide an appropriate level of reassurance and information if this is asked of you. Finally, you should try to effect a proper closure to the interview, particularly in an OSCE. Consider using phrases such as: "Is there anything we discussed that wasn't entirely clear?" or "Are there any further questions you would like me to answer?" to round off your history. With such questions, it is preferable to put the emphasis on whether or not *you* made it clear enough to the patient rather than whether *they* were able to understand the information.

The structure of these scenarios can easily be used to develop an appropriate approach to the OSLER (and other similar medical examinations), which is used in some medical schools alongside the OSCE, either for formative or summative assessment.

A CONTENT GUIDE FOR HISTORY TAKING

The Calgary–Cambridge model incorporates the traditional medical approach (below left). When recording the content of the medical interview, consider the adapted model on the right, which is based on the Calgary–Cambridge model, as proposed by Silverman et al.

Traditional medical approach	Non-traditional approach
The history	**Adapted Calgary–Cambridge framework** Patient's problem list **1.** **2.**
Presenting complaint	**Exploration of patient's problems**
History of presenting complaint	*Medical perspective (disease)* Sequence of events Symptom analysis Relevant systems review
Past medical history	
Drug and allergy history	*Patient's perspective (illness)* Effects on life and feelings Ideas Concerns Expectations
Family history	
Personal and social history	**Background information – context** Past medical history Drug and allergy history Family history Personal and social history Review of systems
Physical examination	**Physical examination**
Differential diagnosis **Investigations**	**Differential diagnosis/problem list**
Management	**Physician's plan of management** Investigations Treatment alternatives

General OSCE tips

PRACTICE PAST STATIONS WITH A SMALL GROUP OF FRIENDS

- Two to three friends are ideal – one student, one patient and possibly one examiner to note what you have and haven't done well.
- Come up with a list of past stations and potential other stations and test your friends in a pressurised environment to simulate the real thing.
- Watch your friends closely – you will pick up things from others that you wouldn't have thought of yourself.

PRACTICAL REVISION

- Go on the wards to see patients with stomas, fistulas, etc., before your exams – if you haven't seen something before it is usually obvious to the examiner.
- Revising from books and notes should only supplement your practical revision for OSCEs.

USE YOUR READING TIME BEFORE EACH STATION EFFICIENTLY

- Compose yourself and do not dwell on past stations – the great thing about OSCEs is you have a chance to start afresh with a different examiner every station.
- In your reading time, think carefully about what the question is asking you to do, examiners will get annoyed if you do not follow the instructions carefully.
  - Is it a focussed history, examination with a few pertinent questions, examination with no questions allowed or other?
  - If it is an examination have they asked you to only examine one aspect or a complete examination? If in doubt about the instructions, ask the examiner.
- In your reading time, ask yourself what things do you often forget when practicing this type of station so that you can remember it in the real thing.
- In spotter stations (i.e. stations where you are presented with patients who often exhibit pathognomonic signs), your instructions may read along the lines of "Please examine this patient's hand/knee/lower limb, etc., and give your diagnosis..." Use your reading time to come up with potential diagnoses you might see when you walk in to prevent yourself drawing a blank as you walk in.

WASH YOUR HANDS BEFORE AND AFTER SEEING EACH PATIENT/SIMULATED PATIENT

- Practice doing this before each station and make sure you point out to your friends when they have failed to do so. Hand hygiene is very important and students may be marked down for a failure to comply with this.

BE FRIENDLY TO YOUR EXAMINERS

- Smile and make eye contact with your examiners.
- They are more likely to be communicative with you if you are communicative with them.

BE FRIENDLY TO YOUR PATIENTS

- Take time to introduce yourself to the patient and establish some rapport (if they like you, they may even end up helping you along the way).
- When allowed to ask questions, be sure to ask how their condition has affected them and their activities of daily living.

DO NOT PANIC IN TRICKY STATIONS

- If you find a station challenging, it is likely others will find it hard too. Reassure yourself that it is challenging not because of your performance being poor but because the examiner wishes to assess your skills under pressure. Think of these stations as opportunities to gain extra marks as many students will freeze in these stations.

TIPS FROM EXPERIENCED EXAMINERS

FORGET ABOUT YOUR PREVIOUS STATION

- Remember, each station is completely separate and provides a fresh start.
- No one knows how well you did in the past station (including yourself and your next examiner) so put it out of your mind and focus on the next station.
- The only way the examiner may think you have performed poorly generally is by your demeanour if you let a "bad" station affect you.

PROFESSIONALISM IS IMPORTANT

- Treat each patient/simulated patient with respect and use eye contact.
- Do not just spend time looking at paper/results – if there is a patient/simulated patient, you are expected to act professionally as you would in reality.

LOOK AROUND FOR CLUES IN EACH STATION

- Disease identifiers, e.g. walking aids, inhalers, oxygen, cardiac monitors, insulin pumps.
- Are there any props lying around – if so, use them as it is likely to be on the examiner's marking criteria!

IF IN DOUBT ABOUT WHAT IS EXPECTED OF YOU, SEEK CLARIFICATION

- Examiners want you to pass and will usually try to point you in the right direction.
- The worst that can happen is they will say "do as you see fit."
- An example for when you might seek clarification – You are told to examine the "chest" (usually synonymous with a respiratory examination) but see a sternotomy scar. Point out that you see the sternotomy scar which would most likely indicate coronary artery bypass grafting or a valve replacement and ask if they would like you to conduct a cardiovascular examination or a respiratory examination.

TALK TO YOUR EXAMINER UNLESS INSTRUCTED NOT TO DO SO

- Most examiners like students to talk through what they are doing as they go along.
- It helps the examiner to signpost things that are paramount to the station.
- Some examiners may ask you not to talk as you go along and prefer you to simply present at the end. If this happens, do not be put off by this.

Tips for approaching a history-taking OSCE station

THE START

- **Greetings** – Greet the patient with a smile and do not rush your introduction.
- **Opening statement** – Always start with an open question and do not interrupt their opening gambit.
- **Negotiate/confirm the agenda** – After acknowledging the patient's problems brought up by their opening statement, screen for other problems (e.g. "I'm sorry to hear you've been having difficulty with X, before we go into that further can I ask if there are any other problems you've noticed or would like to discuss?").
- **Good communication skills** – Even in what may feel like a contrived or unreal situation, it is important to show the patient that you are listening empathetically to their problems and concerns.
- **ABCDE approach** – You may be required to start with an ABCDE approach if the patient appears critically unwell (i.e. peri-arrest/unable to give a history). Read the station's instructions here carefully. *If the instructions ask you to take a history and the patient is well enough to do so, then you should proceed as such and not go to the ABCDE approach.* If in doubt, you could do a streamlined ABC check and then proceed to the history.

THE MIDDLE

- **Have a system** – If facing an unfamiliar station, consider adopting a basic framework such as SOCRATES – this will show the examiner you are thinking systematically.
- **History of presenting complaint** – This is the most important part of most histories and you should aim to spend roughly half of the allocated time addressing this.
- **Summarise when stuck** – Not only can this buy you some time to think of your next move, it also comforts the patient and examiner by letting them know you have been listening and may also elucidate any area that was unclear.
- **Respond to cues** – Do not ignore cues, both verbal and non-verbal. You have your agenda, but so does the patient. Simulated patients (SPs) will often try and point you in the right direction if you let them. Let them air their concerns as they arise and do not ignore them (you can always acknowledge them and signpost them for later if you feel necessary). Acknowledge and legitimise them, answer them to the best of your ability and come back to them later in the history to see if their concerns have changed at all.
- **Ideas, concerns and expectations** – You will be expected to not only ask about the patient's perspective in their illness but also fully explore it to gain the top marks; in the modern consultation it is important that you listen to the patient's concerns attentively – this may even help prompt you down a line of questioning.
- **Review of systems** – This can be helpful if after the history of presenting complaint you are still very unclear as to possible diagnoses. It may help you realise that you have been

"barking up the wrong tree" entirely and help you shift the focus of the history before it is too late. Start with an open question e.g. "Have you noticed any other symptoms?" Then move on to closed relevant system-based questions. If given a positive answer, you should then direct further questions towards this symptom.

- **Communication skills** – Taking a history is not a tick box exercise; remember to use good communication skills e.g. mirroring, empathy, active listening, signposting and summarising.

THE END

- **To finish** – At the end of every history, summarise and ask the patient if you have missed anything or if they have any questions/concerns you haven't already answered.
- **Differential diagnosis** – Top marks for a history often come at the end with how you present your working diagnosis and differentials.
- **Investigations and management** – The investigations and management listed in this book are designed to cover the most likely differentials; they are not necessarily comprehensive, nor do they all need to be utilised in every case (in an exam, you should only say the relevant ones to the scenario you are presented with if/when asked by the examiner).

KNOWLEDGE

- A good understanding of the NICE guidelines on cancer referrals can be useful in constructing your histories and remembering the important red flags to ask in each history. These can be found online:
  https://www.nice.org.uk/guidance/ng12/chapter/1-Recommendations-organised-by-site-of-cancer
- NICE also have many useful clinical knowledge summaries that are designed with primary care physicians in mind. They provide succinct summaries of the best available evidence and guidance on a multitude of different problems seen in general practice as well as on the wards. These are referred to throughout this book in the "Further Reading" sections and can be found online: http://cks.nice.org.uk/#?char=A

USING THIS BOOK TO PREPARE FOR YOUR OSCE – FOCUS YOUR HISTORY

As you can see by looking at "OSCE marking scheme – Manchester Medical School (pp. xli)" being awarded a good mark is not simply reliant on asking every question pertaining to a given history. A lot of the criteria relate to your communication skills and the structure of the consultation.

In the OSCE, you are unlikely to be able to ask all the questions listed in each history in this book. Aim to spend most of your allocated time focussing on the important parts of the history to come to your diagnosis, whilst at the same time ruling out red flags and considering the patient's perspective. Don't spend a long time going through the background information (i.e. PMH, DH, FH, SH) as it often won't add as much as the medical and patient's perspectives. In an OSCE, the patients are usually well rehearsed to give you the background information quickly with a simple single open question.

Example history – Knee pain

This example history shows a logical way a history station could be approached in an OSCE using the Calgary–Cambridge *process* to gain the content of the traditional medical history. This section will focus on structure, giving example dialogue and a full breakdown of the history. This example gives all the information that might be expected of a candidate. Usually, the OSCE instructions will be to focus on one element of the session e.g. the history itself. In a time-limited scenario, it may not be possible to go through all the individual points this example touches on. In this case, it is important that sufficient time is allocated to each area the OSCE instructions are examining you on in order to satisfy picking up marks in each area.

Histories for specific presenting complaints elsewhere in this book will focus on the *content* to be obtained by the medical student, rather than the strict process and exact dialogue. They will therefore not focus on the communication skills aspect in detail. In order to obtain the content however, a similar *process* should be used by the student/doctor as shown in this example history.

INITIATING THE SESSION

1. Greet the patient, introduce yourself and explain the reason for the interview

    Doctor: *Hello, is it Mrs Susan Smith?*
    Patient: *Yes, please call me Sue.*
    Doctor: *Hi Sue, my name is Joe Bloggs. I am a junior doctor at the practice. Can I just confirm your date of birth?*
    Patient: *25th December, 1945.*
    Doctor: *It's nice to meet you Sue. I understand you've been having some pain; I'd like to ask a few questions to try to get to the bottom of the issue if that is OK.*
    Patient: *Of course.*

2. Open question

    Doctor: *Can you tell me more about this pain you've had?*
    Patient: *I've had this terrible pain in my knees now for the last year or so, but it seems to be getting worse. I've tried all kinds of things for it, but nothing seems to work. It's got to the extent where I'm struggling going for walks with my friends now *CUE*. I spoke to my sister who told me it could be something serious *CUE*, so I thought I'd get it checked out.*

3. Screen for other problems

> **Doctor:** *I'm sorry to hear that it's stopping you going for walks with your friends; before we talk further about that, can I just check if there are any other problems you wished to discuss today?*
>
> **Patient:** *No, I just want to find out what is causing this pain.*

> The patient's opening gambit included several **cues** (her walking and her sister's concerns as well as her own concerns). Before moving on to the screen for other problems in this case, it is necessary to **acknowledge** the problems and concerns she has mentioned and show empathy so that it doesn't look like you are simply ignoring them. On screening for other problems, the patient has given an **expectation** for the interview.

GATHERING INFORMATION – THE MEDICAL PERSPECTIVE

1. Ask further open questions to determine a timeline of events

> **Doctor:** *Ok, can you tell me how the pain began?*
>
> **Patient:** *It seemed to just creep up on me. I first noticed when I was bending down or going up the stairs about a year ago. Recently though it just seems to be getting worse; it is there all the time and really affects my walking *CUE*.*

2. Explore cues

> **Doctor:** *Tell me about your walking*
>
> **Patient:** *Since my husband Paul died 2 years ago, the only regular interaction I get is when I go walking with my friends Sanjay and Monica. They were good friends with Paul and I and don't mind when I tell them stories about Paul's younger days. We go for a walk around the local park every week, but recently I've had to cancel on them and have been a bit lonely.*
>
> **Doctor:** *I'm really sorry to hear that. Shall we see if we can get to the bottom of the pain and hopefully then we can get you back out walking again.*

3. Symptom analysis

> **Doctor:** *You mentioned the pain is there all the time. Is it worse any particular time of the day?*
> **Patient:** *It seems to be quite bad at night.*
> **Doctor:** *What does it feel like?*
> **Patient:** *It is an aching pain really. It seems to get worse when I'm walking.*
> **Doctor:** *Does anything else make it better or worse?*
> **Patient:** *Not that I have noticed.*
> **Doctor:** *What have you tried to help the pain? Have you taken any pain killers?*
> **Patient:** *I've been taking paracetamol regularly, but it doesn't seem to touch it.*
> **Doctor:** *Is the pain just in your knees or does it go anywhere else?*
> **Patient:** *Only in my knees.*
> **Doctor:** *Is the pain worse in either knee?*
> **Patient:** *It is about the same in each knee I think.*
> **Doctor:** *Have you ever injured your knees?*
> **Patient:** *No.*

The mnemonic "SOCRATES" can be useful when taking a history of someone's pain:

Site
Onset
Character
Radiation
Associated features
Timing
Exacerbating/relieving factors
Severity

4. Relevant systems review

Doctor: *Have you noticed any other symptoms?*
Patient: *I don't think so.*
Doctor: *Do your knees ever swell up?*
Patient: *Now that you mention it, yes they do. Sometimes they're like balloons.*
Doctor: *Do they seem stiff first thing in the morning?*
Patient: *Not that I have noticed.*
Doctor: *Do you get pain in any of your other joints?*
Patient: *Yes, I've been getting similar pains in my hips and in my neck for a few years, but they don't really bother me.*

5. Summarise

Doctor: *So you've been having pain in both your knees for a year now. It came on gradually, but now is constant and has gotten to the extent where it has stopped you going for walks with your friends. You've tried taking paracetamol, but that doesn't help it. You've never injured your knees. They can swell up, but don't feel particularly stiff. You've also been getting similar pains in your hips and neck, but aren't as concerned about them. Have I missed anything?*

GATHERING INFORMATION – THE PATIENT'S PERSPECTIVE

1. Effects on life & feelings

Doctor: *You mentioned it has stopped you going for walks. How else has it affected you?*
Patient: *I have been struggling to do my shopping. I have even been having some difficulty getting washed in the morning.*
Doctor: *I'm sorry to hear that. I hope you don't mind me commenting, but it seems to have affected your mood somewhat. Would you agree?*
Patient: *It really has doctor. I don't feel depressed, but I am fed up now.*

2. Explore ideas

Doctor: *Have you got any ideas yourself regarding what might be causing this pain?*
Patient: *Well my sister thought it could be cancer.*
Doctor: *Is that something you think it could be?*

Patient: *Not really, but it scared me enough to make me come in. I thought it was just old age.*
Doctor: *What is it about your symptoms that makes your sister worry about it being cancer?*
Patient: *She knew someone who's child had some leg pains and it turned out to be cancer.*
Doctor: *Just to set your mind at rest, it doesn't sound like cancer to me, but we can talk more about that in a little bit.*

Notice the patient in this instance initially gives her *sister's* idea and not her own. In this case you can glean more information by asking about her own ideas and checking if they marry up with her sister's ideas. This is something patients commonly do in practice even though their own ideas are often very different.

3. Explore concerns

Doctor: *Is there anything else you are concerned could be causing the pain?*
Patient: *I don't think so.*
Doctor: *Is there anything in general that is concerning you?*
Patient: *Just that I might not be able to join my friends on their walks anymore really.*

4. Explore expectations

Doctor: *Would I be right in thinking the reason you have come in today is to find out what is causing the pain and to try and get you back walking?*
Patient: *That would be excellent doctor.*
Doctor: *Was there anything else you were hoping for?*
Patient: *No, that is about it.*

Exploring patient's ideas, concerns and expectations can seem robotic if simply using it as a tick box exercise. This example shows how you can use your communication skills to test a hypothesis regarding the patient's expectations. If doing this, you should seek to confirm whether the patient had any other additional expectations.

BACKGROUND INFORMATION

1. Past medical history

Doctor: *Do you suffer from any other medical conditions?*
Patient: *Just blood pressure.*

2. Drug and allergy history

Doctor: *Do you take any medications?*
Patient: *Yes, here is my list.*
Doctor: *Do you have any allergies?*
Patient: *No.*

3. Family history

Doctor: *Has anyone in your family suffered from similar problems?*
Patient: *No.*

4. Personal and social history

Doctor: *Do you drink alcohol?*
Patient: *Only on special occasions.*
Doctor: *Have you ever smoked?*
Patient: *No.*
Doctor: *Are you retired or still working?*
Patient: *Retired.*
Doctor: *What was your occupation before you retired?*
Patient: *I was a housewife.*

PHYSICAL EXAMINATION (*IF ASKED FOR IN OSCE INSTRUCTIONS*)

Physical examination is not covered in this book in order to focus on the history-taking element of the consultation. Please consider a relevant textbook such as *The Easy Guide to OSCEs for Specialities* and *The Easy Guide to OSCEs for Final Year Medical Students* by Akunjee et al. for a guide to examination in OSCEs.

EXPLANATION AND PLANNING (*IF ASKED FOR IN OSCE INSTRUCTIONS*)

1. Working diagnosis related to the patient's own ideas and concerns

Doctor: *You mentioned earlier you thought it was due to old age. This is partly true. I think the pain you are suffering is due to wear and tear in the joints, commonly known as "arthritis." What do you know about arthritis?*
Patient: *Oh, I know about arthritis. Its where you get pains in your joints from old age.*
Doctor: *That's about right, it is more common as we get older, but there are things we can do to help it. It can also cause pain in other joints including the hips and neck.*

2. Shared decision-making (investigations and management)

Patient: *Do I need an x-ray or something?*
Doctor: *We don't always do x-rays initially. We often try to treat it first using simple measures such as pain killers and gels, as well as exercise and weight loss, which has been shown to be the best non-surgical management option. If things don't improve and are still affecting your life, then we often use x-rays to guide further management such as surgery if necessary. How do you feel about this? How would you like to manage the condition?*
Patient: *As long as there is something out there that can help me, I'll try anything.*
Doctor: *OK, well we could try an anti-inflammatory gel, ibuprofen. How does that sound?*
Patient: *Excellent.*
Doctor: *Can I just double check you have had no problems with anti-inflammatory medications before?*
Patient: *I have had them before and been fine. What are the side effects?*
Doctor: *It is usually well tolerated when used as a gel, but can cause skin irritation, indigestion and allergic reactions rarely.*

The amount of information you give in this section should depend on what the OSCE instructions state. If they only ask you to take a history, then little if any explanation and planning needs to discussed with the patient (the examiner however may ask you questions at the end of the history).

CLOSING THE SESSION

1. Summary

Doctor: *So to summarise, we have discussed about your knee pain, which you have been concerned about as it has stopped you going for walks with your friends as well as causing difficulty doing your shopping. We discussed about arthritis, which is due to wear and tear as you thought was most likely yourself. You are happy to try a gel for your knees in the first instance and we discussed how exercise and weight loss can also help. Do you have any remaining questions or concerns I haven't answered for you that you'd like to go over?*

Patient: *No thank you.*

2. Contract – safety netting and follow-up

Doctor: *OK, well in that case, what I'd suggest is if the pain doesn't get any better in the next few months or you feel it is still stopping you from getting out on your walks then please come back and see me and we can discuss any other options. How does that sound?*

Patient: *That sounds wonderful, thank you doctor.*

OSCE marking scheme – Manchester Medical School

Manchester Medical School is one of the many medical schools that routinely use OSCEs as part of their examination process. OSCEs are an excellent method of examination as they:

- Eliminate examiner bias as far as is possible for a clinical examination that has to be assessed by a clinician
- Test a breadth of knowledge and skills
- Mimic the real clinical situation in outpatients and GP surgeries where most medicine nowadays is undertaken
- Provide a time limit to your consultation that is comparable to the time doctors have to assess and manage their patients in practice

The Manchester OSCE consists of 16 stations, each lasting 9 minutes (8 minutes + 1 minute preparation). Each station is designed to test specific skills and application of knowledge. The skills tested include:

- History taking
- Communication skills
- Examination of different systems
- Interpretation of images (e.g. x-rays)
- Interpretation of data
- Practical procedures
- Management of ethical dilemmas

CLINICAL INFORMATION

The examiner has access to the patient clinical information to allow the examiner to mark the medical student against the marking criteria. The clinical information may include:

- Key points in history
- Onset of symptoms
- Duration
- Other symptoms
- Patient's ideas, concerns and expectations
- Feelings and effect of symptoms on patient's life
- Past medical problems
- Any treatment given to date for this problem
- Regular medications and drug allergies
- Relevant family, personal and social history

THE MARKING SCHEME

Below are different sections of the standardised Manchester Medical School marking scheme relating to history taking. These have been taken from the manchester.ac.uk domain with permission. The link below also provides access to the examiner training implemented in order to facilitate use of the marking scheme as well as standardising the OSCE across the different sites of the large medical school. When preparing for your OSCE, it would be wise to have this marking scheme in mind. If practicing in groups of three or more, the "examiner" should use this marking scheme to provide relevant structured feedback.

Reference: http://sites.mms.manchester.ac.uk/prime/osce/newmarking/

OVERALL CONDUCT OF THE CONSULTATION

- Candidate introduces self, states role and checks the patient's identity (Name and DOB)
- Explains the purpose of consultation
- Keeps the patient's confidentiality, safety and dignity foremost
- Seeks consent
- Maintains a courteous and caring demeanour
- Listens attentively and acts with empathy, honesty and sensitivity
- Demonstrates a fluent, coherent and confident approach
- Considers patient's preferences and makes no attempt to force or coerce patient
- Manages time and closes appropriately, thanking the patient
- Dresses appropriately

HISTORY-TAKING SKILLS

- Uses a structured, fluent and focussed approach
- Uses a combination of open questions and closed questions
- Responds to information given by patient, rather than appearing to follow a set formula of questions
- Obtains key and relevant information and shows the ability to use the information
- Elicits and acknowledges the patient's ideas, concerns and expectations
- Discovers the impact of the problem on the patient's life
- Repeats, reflects, summarises and clarifies
- Avoids premature or false reassurance

> You can see the marking scheme closely mirrors the Calgary–Cambridge model. An emphasis is placed on a fluid interaction with the patient rather than simply following a rigid approach. A true understanding of the Calgary–Cambridge model facilitates a process that is more fluid than the traditional medical model approach.

NON-VERBAL COMMUNICATION

- Establishes a rapport early and maintains it
- Maintains a positive and open body language and eye contact
- Maintains a calm and composed demeanour

- Responds to cues and follows up appropriately
- Uses or offers appropriate and understandable visual methods for conveying information e.g. diagrams if applicable
- Uses appropriate seating position

CLINICAL KNOWLEDGE AND DIAGNOSIS

- Questioning, where applicable, indicates the depth of understanding of the clinical condition/pathology
- Identifies and recognises the underlying problem
- Interprets the data or information provided, in the context of the problem, in order to come to a conclusion
- Integrates the information gathered
- Applies knowledge to the patient's current problem
- Generates a plausible list of differential diagnoses based on the information gathered
- Is able to propose, justify and defend their diagnosis or differential diagnosis

A mark is given for each section on a five-point scale from "uses no elements" to "uses all the elements." Examiners use this marking scheme to help them make a global judgement about the student's overall competence on the station, based on a seven-point scale (with four and above).

General medicine and geriatrics

1

TIRED ALL THE TIME

INITIATING THE SESSION

- Greet the patient, ask an open question and screen for other problems

MEDICAL PERSPECTIVE

SEQUENCE OF EVENTS

- **Open question** – Can you tell me more about what's been going on? What exactly do you mean when you say you feel tired/fatigued?
- **Timeline** – When did you first notice this? How has it progressed?

SYMPTOM ANALYSIS

- **Ideas/pointers** – Can you think of any reason for feeling tired?
- **Sleep** – How are you sleeping? Does sleep refresh you?
- **Timing** – Do you ever not feel tired? *If so*, when?
- **Exacerbating/relieving factors** – Does anything worsen your tiredness? (e.g. exercise, emotional stress)
- **Other symptoms** – How have you been feeling otherwise? Have you had any other symptoms?

SYSTEMS REVIEW/DIRECT QUESTIONING

- **Fever** – Have you been feeling feverish or generally unwell? *If so*, in what way?
- **Viral illness** – Have you had a sore throat or a cold recently?
- **Cancer** – Have you noticed a cough? Change in bowel habit? Any lumps? Problems urinating? Have you noticed any change in your weight over the past few months? *If so*, was this intentional or not? How is your appetite?

RED FLAGS

Weight loss
Change in bowel habit
Dysphagia
Cough >3 weeks
Bleeding (e.g. haematuria)
Breast lump

- **Hypothyroidism** – Do you find yourself feeling cold even when others say it is warm?
- **Diabetes** – Do you have to go to the toilet more often recently? Do you find yourself feeling constantly thirsty despite drinking more than you used to?
- **Depression** – Have you been suffering from low mood recently? *If so,* for how long? Do you have any hobbies you enjoy doing?
- **Chronic fatigue syndrome/fibromyalgia** – Do you have any pain in your muscles? Headaches? How is your memory and concentration?
- **Menorrhagia (anaemia)** – Do you suffer from heavy periods?

PATIENT'S PERSPECTIVE

- **Effect on life** – How has your tiredness affected your daily life?
- **Feelings** – How do you feel about it?
- **Ideas** – What do you think is causing your tiredness?
- **Concerns** – Are you concerned anything else could be causing it? Is there anything in general that is concerning you?
- **Expectations** – Other than getting to the bottom of the tiredness, was there anything in particular you were hoping for when you made this appointment?

BACKGROUND INFORMATION

PMH

- Do you suffer from any medical or psychiatric conditions?
- *Ask specifically about diabetes and any past history of malignancy*

DH

- Are you taking any medications? Have any of these been changed recently?
- Are you taking any over-the-counter medications? Do you have any allergies?

FH

- Do any conditions run in your family?
- *Ask specifically about diabetes, thyroid disease and malignancy*

SH

- Are you working presently? *If so,* what is your job? What does that involve? Has your problem affected your job in any way?
- Can you tell me about your home situation (*occupants and any difficulties*)? How is your problem affecting your home life?
- Do you smoke? (*Number of packets a day x years smoked = "pack-years" which approximates to the total cigarette consumption*)
- Do you drink alcohol? *If so,* how much do you drink in a week?

CLOSING THE SESSION

- summary ± examination/explanation and planning/contract

> **IMPORTANT POINTS**
> - Be empathetic to the patient's concerns and how the symptoms have affected them. Communication skills are vital in histories like this one, and marks are likely to be awarded for gaining a true appreciation of how the problem has affected the patient.
> - In this history the cause will often be a non-sinister one; however, you are unlikely to be awarded top marks unless you have been seen to actively be ruling out other causes.

DIFFERENTIAL DIAGNOSIS

ENVIRONMENTAL (MOST COMMON)

- Poor sleeping environment or an unstructured sleeping routine
- Working long hours with stressful jobs ("burnout")
- Having small children and/or being a carer for someone

CANCER (MOST SERIOUS)

- Constitutional symptoms such as weight loss, decreased appetite and fever
- The big four causes of cancer are breast, prostate, lung and colorectal carcinomas
- Suspect in patients with significant weight loss, symptoms and risk factors for a particular cancer (e.g. suspect lung cancer in a patient with haemoptysis and breathlessness, who has smoked for 40 years)

VIRAL ILLNESS (NON-SPECIFIC)

- Short history of flu-like symptoms that if left a week will disappear by itself
- More severe cases can result in a prolonged post-viral state of fatigue (*see also chronic fatigue syndrome below*)

INFECTIOUS MONONUCLEOSIS

- The "kissing disease" is caused by Epstein–Barr virus (suspect in adolescents)
- History of sore throat and flu-like symptoms that persist longer than would be expected from other common viruses

ANAEMIA

- Blood loss is the most common cause of a microcytic anaemia – remember to consider NSAIDs, menorrhagia and colorectal carcinoma as likely underlying causes
- Chronic disease can cause a normocytic picture (anaemia of chronic disease)
- Folate/B12 deficiency, hypothyroidism and alcoholism can cause a macrocytic picture

HYPOTHYROIDISM

- Weight gain despite decreased appetite, intolerance of cold, constipation, menstrual irregularities, low mood and feeling slow are amongst many features
- There may be a family history of thyroid disease or just autoimmune disease
- Usually female and middle-aged

DIABETES MELLITUS

- Polyuria, polydipsia, increased appetite and weight loss
- Presentation with tiredness is most commonly seen in type I – usually a young adolescent presenting for the first time but can also be a known type 1 diabetic who is not taking his/her insulin
- Type II can also present with fatigue, but is much more likely than type I to be asymptomatic

CARDIAC, RENAL OR LIVER FAILURE

- Ankle oedema and symptoms specific to the failing system
- Past history of cardiac, renal or liver disease is likely to be present

DEPRESSION

- Core symptoms – low mood, anhedonia and fatigue present for >2 weeks
- Typical symptoms – sleep disturbance, early morning waking (>2 hours earlier than usual), decreased appetite and weight loss (>10%)

CHRONIC FATIGUE SYNDROME

- Persistent fatigue for >6 months in a previously healthy individual that is not due to physical exertion, not relieved by rest and can't be explained by a medical condition
- Myalgia, headaches, sore throat and poor concentration and memory
- There may be a past history of irritable bowel syndrome and/or fibromyalgia

IATROGENIC

- Many medications can cause fatigue (particularly beta-blockers) – ask if any medications have been changed recently

INVESTIGATIONS

- Cardio-respiratory examination and breast/PR examination (if breast/colorectal cancer suspected)
- Check for a palpable thyroid
- FBC, U&Es, LFTs, TFTs, blood glucose, ESR and CRP
- Urinalysis for diabetes and renal failure
- Monospot test for infectious mononucleosis
- Serum ferritin/B12/folate if evidence of anaemia

- Upper and/or lower GIT investigations if unexplained iron deficiency anaemia
- Based on clinical suspicion – Mammography/USS and biopsy for breast cancer; PSA for prostatic cancer; chest x-ray and bronchoscopy for lung cancer; faecal occult blood and colonoscopy for colorectal cancer

MANAGEMENT

- **Personal circumstances** – Sleep hygiene (a structured sleeping routine); can work situation be altered? Would counselling be beneficial?
- **Virus/infectious mononucleosis** – Bed rest and hydration
- **Anaemia** – Treat depending on cause
- **Hypothyroidism** – Thyroxine
- **Diabetes mellitus type 1** – Insulin therapy (consider insulin pump if poorly controlled); type II – appropriate diabetic medication and/or insulin
- **Cancer** – Refer onwards for specialist management
- **Cardiac, renal or liver failure** – Treat depending on cause
- **Depression** – SSRIs and CBT
- **Chronic fatigue syndrome** – Non-vigorous exercise (excessive exercise will exacerbate the condition) and CBT

FURTHER READING

NICE CKS on tiredness, http://cks.nice.org.uk/tirednessfatigue-in-adults

FALLS

INITIATING THE SESSION

- Greet the patient, ask an open question and screen for other problems

MEDICAL PERSPECTIVE

SEQUENCE OF EVENTS AND SYMPTOM ANALYSIS

Before

- **Open question** – Can you talk me through what happened exactly? What were you doing at the time? What do you think caused you to fall?
- **Clarify** – Did you have a fall or did you collapse unexpectedly? *If collapse, go to collapse and seizures history, pp. 61*
- **Aura** – How did you feel immediately before the episode? Did you have any warning that something was about to happen?
- **Screen for serious causes** – Did you have any chest pain at the time? Any shortness of breath? Any palpitations?
- **Screen for prior illness** – Have you been unwell recently?
- **Environmental** – Did you trip over anything or slip?

During

- **Fall** – How did you fall exactly? Did you hit your head?
- **LOC** – Did you lose consciousness? *If so*, for how long? Do you remember everything that happened?
- **Witness** – Did anyone witness the episode? How did they describe it? Did you have a fit? *If so, see collapse and seizures history, pp. 61*

After

- **Injury** – How did you feel after the fall? Did you hurt yourself anywhere? Have you been able to walk since the fall?
- **Previous falls** – Have you suffered from falls before? *If so*, how many and when? What happened those times?
- **Eyesight** – How is your eyesight? Do you have difficulty getting about?

SYSTEMS REVIEW

- **Constitutional** – Have you noticed any significant weight loss recently? Any night sweats? Any lumps anywhere? Any fever?
- **RS/CVS** – Have you noticed a cough? Any shortness of breath? Any chest pain?
- **GUT** – Have you noticed any pain when passing urine? Increased frequency? Any blood in the urine?
- **GIT** – Have you had any abdominal pain recently? How have your bowels been? Any bleeding from the back passage?

PATIENT'S PERSPECTIVE

- **Effect on life** – How have your fall(s) affected your daily life?
- **Feelings** – How do you feel about what happened?

- **Ideas** – What do you think caused you to fall?
- **Concerns** – Are you concerned anything else caused the fall? Is there anything in general that is concerning you?
- **Expectations** – When you made the appointment, other than getting my opinion, did you have any particular hopes or expectations?

BACKGROUND INFORMATION

PMH

- Do you suffer from any medical conditions?

DH

- Are you taking any medications? Have any been changed or added recently?
- *Ask specifically about aspirin, warfarin and other anti-platelet/anti-coagulants as well as any anti-hypertensives and sedatives*
- Any allergies?

FH

- Do any conditions run in your family?

SH

- Can you tell me about your home situation (*occupants and any difficulties*)? How is your problem affecting your home life? Who is at home with you?
- How is your mobility? Do you need any walking aids?
- Do you have stairs?
- Have you had any modifications put in place such as rails or a chair lift?
- Do you have any carers?
- Do you have any family or friends that are able to help with things like shopping? Who prepares your meals?
- Are you still working or retired? *If retired,* do you have any particular hobbies? What affect has your falls had on these hobbies?
- How much alcohol do you drink? Had you been drinking at the time of your fall?
- Do you smoke?

CLOSING THE SESSION

- summary ± examination/explanation and planning/contract

> **IMPORTANT POINTS**
>
> - It is very important to distinguish between a mechanical fall and a collapse. If the patient has collapsed, a more detailed history around this is required to discover the cause of the collapse *(see collapse and seizures history, pp. 61)*
> - The patient's perspective and the social aspect of a falls history is critical. Elderly patients presenting with falls may well be struggling to cope with other aspects of daily life
> - Always consider the damage the fall has done as well – did they hit their head and is there any indication of trauma elsewhere?

DIFFERENTIAL DIAGNOSIS

The aetiology of a fall is often multifactorial in elderly patients. Poor eyesight, poor mobility, poor cognition, a patient's environment and lack of support can all make a patient more susceptible to having falls. Simple measures should be taken to help prevent falls e.g. ensuring their home environment is safe and suitable for them.

MECHANICAL FALL (MOST COMMON)

- No red flags to indicate other conditions; good recollection of fall
- If loss of consciousness (LOC), collaborative history reveals this was due to the fall itself
- History of similar falls; usually elderly and frail
- Poor eyesight, mobility and cognition all contribute
- May trip over loose carpets, wires, objects on floor etc.

POSTURAL HYPOTENSION

- Often after the patient moves from a lying/sitting position to standing
- Very brief episode (lasting a few seconds) following a "head rush" or unsteadiness
- Anti-cholinergic medications e.g. tricyclic anti-depressants or anti-hypertensive medications may contribute

INVESTIGATIONS

- Full cardiovascular and neurological examination
- Assess gait, balance, vision, cognition and risk of osteoporosis
- Bloods – FBC, U&Es and inflammatory markers if underlying illness suspected
- ECG if there is a lack of clarity or the patient cannot give a reliable history of the fall
- Lying and standing blood pressure – Drop of >20/10 mm Hg = postural hypotension

MANAGEMENT

- Avoid precipitating factors (e.g. tell patients to get up slowly and carefully)
- Involve social workers and occupational therapists
- Referral to a falls clinic (usually run by geriatricians)
- Ensure the patient's home environment is safe – consider rails, chair lifts or even moving to sheltered accommodation
- Review medication – Do they need to be on all their tablets?
- Strength and balance training

REFERENCE

1. NICE head injury guidance, https://www.nice.org.uk/guidance/cg176

FURTHER READING

NICE CKS on falls, http://cks.nice.org.uk/falls-risk-assessment

PYREXIA (ADULTS)

INITIATING THE SESSION

- Greet the patient, ask an open question and screen for other problems

MEDICAL PERSPECTIVE

SEQUENCE OF EVENTS AND SYMPTOM ANALYSIS

- **Clarify** – What exactly do you mean when you say you feel feverish?
- **Timeline** – Can you tell me how your illness started from the beginning?
- **Other symptoms** – How are you feeling generally? Any nausea? Pain anywhere? Any night sweats? *Clarify dates*
- **Timing** – When does the fever tend to come on? How often?

SYSTEMS REVIEW

NB: These are screening questions; if a positive answer is given to any of them, it necessitates further probing about the symptom in question

- **Constitutional** – Have you lost any weight recently? How is your appetite? Have you travelled anywhere abroad recently? Any insect bites?
- **Haematological** – Have you been bruising or bleeding more easily? Getting recurrent infections? Been more tired than normal?
- **RS/CVS** – Have you had a cough? Any sputum? Any blood? Any chest pain?
- **GIT** – Have you had any change in bowel habit? Diarrhoea or vomiting?
- **GUT** – Do you have any pain on urination? Are you going more frequently? Any blood in your urine? Have you recently had unprotected sex with a new partner?
- **NS** – Do you have a headache? Neck stiffness? A rash?
- **Breast** – Have you noticed any lumps or changes in your breasts?
- **MSK** – Are any of your joints or muscles stiff or painful? Any skin lesions or ulcers? Dry eyes or dry mouth? Do your hands change colour in the cold?

> **RED FLAGS**
>
> Weight loss
> Drenching night sweats
> Bleeding/bruising tendency
> New onset anaemia
> Neck stiffness/
>   photophobia
> Non-blanching rash
> Foreign travel

PATIENT PERSPECTIVE

- **Feelings and effect on life** – Has the fever affected your life in any way?
- **Ideas** – Do you have any ideas yourself about what could be causing the fever?
- **Concerns** – Is there anything else you are concerned could be causing it? Is there anything in general that is worrying you?
- **Expectations** – I understand you have come here to get my medical advice, but was there anything you had in mind that you were hoping for when you came here today?

PMH

- Do you have any medical conditions?
- *Ask specifically about HIV, previous malignancy, inflammatory conditions and recent surgery?*

DH

- Are you on any medications? *If so,* have any changed recently? Any allergies?

FH

- Do any conditions run in the family?
- *Ask specifically about autoimmune disease and malignancy?*
- Have any friends or family been unwell recently?

SH

- Are you working presently? *If so,* what is your job? What does that involve? Has your problem affected your job in any way?
- Can you tell me about your home situation (*occupants and any difficulties*)? How is your problem affecting your home life?
- Do you smoke (*have you ever smoked/quantify*)?
- Do you drink alcohol? How much do you drink in a week?

CLOSING THE SESSION

- summary ± examination/explanation and planning/contract

IMPORTANT POINTS

- This would be a tricky station to face in an OSCE, as fever is a non-specific symptom; the initial approach should be to gather a timeline of symptoms and then to systematically search for a cause, making it clear you are ruling out sinister causes such as malignancy and serious infections (e.g. meningitis)
- Start by asking one or two open questions so you can get as much information from them as possible, but direct questioning with closed questions will then be important, particularly in the time-pressurised scenario of an OSCE
- It is important in such a station that you make it clear to the examiner that you are systematically ruling out many different causes – even if you do not get the diagnosis this may be sufficient to impress and gain good marks

DIFFERENTIAL DIAGNOSIS

Fever is normally due to a self-limiting viral infection or uncomplicated bacterial infection. However, where no cause is found after continued fever for 3 weeks despite investigations, pyrexia of unknown origin exists. The causes of this can come under the headings of infection, malignancy or autoimmune as outlined below (the most common of which being infections and malignancy).

INFECTIONS (~1 IN 3 CASES)

TUBERCULOSIS

- Weight loss, night sweats, lymphadenopathy and haemoptysis
- Previous TB exposure; chronic alcoholism, homeless patients, intravenous drug abusers and a compromised immune system are risk factors

ABSCESSES

- There may be no localising symptoms
- Consider intra-abdominal abscess if the patient has had previous abdominal or pelvic surgery, trauma or a history of diverticulosis
- Remember "pus somewhere, pus nowhere, pus under the diaphragm" – Subphrenic abscesses can be hard to diagnose; a high index of suspicion is needed

INFECTIOUS ENDOCARDITIS

- Non-specific malaise and flu-like illness, as well as cardiac and embolic symptoms such as shortness of breath or systemic infarctions
- Classically, patients may have recently been to the dentist where inoculation takes place and/or have pre-existing valvular disease

MALIGNANCY (~1 IN 3 CASES)

- Weight loss and cachexia, as well as other red flags, such as melaena, haemoptysis and haematuria, are likely to be present for specific cancers
- Haematological cancers often present with fever, as well as bruising, recurrent infections and anaemia

AUTOIMMUNE

RHEUMATOID ARTHRITIS

- Symmetrical polyarthritis typically affecting small joints
- Most commonly seen in females
- Hot, swollen and tender joints with morning stiffness

CONNECTIVE TISSUE DISEASE (E.G. SLE)

- Sicca symptoms (e.g. Raynaud's, dry eyes and dry mouth) and fatigue
- Arthralgia, rashes, renal and lung involvement are common amongst CTDs, although any organ can be affected

VASCULITIS

- Skin lesions (possibly necrotic), urticaria, oedema, arthralgia and other systemic features may be present

MISCELLANEOUS

DRUG-INDUCED FEVER

- Some patients have a hypersensitivity to drugs which result in a fever alone rather than anaphylaxis
- Consider this in any patient with no other localising signs or symptoms, who developed fever after starting/increasing the dose of a medication

FAMILIAL MEDITERRANEAN FEVER

- An inherited condition, autosomal recessive, more common in Mediterranean ethnicities, particularly subsets of Jewish communities
- Causes recurrent bouts of fever, abdominal pain and pleuritic chest pain as well as numerous other inflammatory reactions e.g. joint pains

IDIOPATHIC

- In up to 10% of cases no cause will be found

INVESTIGATIONS

- Bloods – FBC, U&Es, LFTs, TFTs, ESR, CRP, serum ferritin and HIV screen
- Autoimmune screen, including rheumatoid factor, ANA and ANCA
- Blood cultures
- Urinalysis; urine microscopy, culture and sensitivity
- Chest x-ray
- Mantoux test and Quantiferon-TB Gold for TB
- CT, MRI or USS depending on suspected malignancy or abscess
- Colonoscopy and upper GIT endoscopy
- Echocardiography
- Doppler

MANAGEMENT

- Tuberculosis is treated using 6 months of isoniazid and rifampicin, with the addition for the first 2 months of pyrazinamide and ethambutol
- Infectious endocarditis – IV gentamicin plus another IV antibiotic (depending on the results of blood cultures and suspected organism)
- Malignancy – Surgery, chemotherapy, radiotherapy and/or palliation
- Rheumatoid arthritis – Methotrexate first-line, with sulphasalazine and leflunomide as second-line therapies; anti-TNF drugs if these fail
- SLE, vasculitis and other autoimmune disorders – Immunosuppressive therapy

FURTHER READING

NICE CKS on TB, http://cks.nice.org.uk/tuberculosis

RASH

INITIATING THE SESSION

- Greet the patient, ask an open question and screen for other problems

MEDICAL PERSPECTIVE

SEQUENCE OF EVENTS

- **Open question** – Can you tell me more about the rash? How did it start?
- **Timeline** – How did it start out? How has it progressed since then?

SYMPTOM ANALYSIS (SOCRATES)

- **Site** – Where exactly is the rash?
- **Onset** – When did it start?
- **Character/colour** – What does it look like?
- **Radiation** – Does it spread anywhere or is it just in one area? *Bilateral versus unilateral*
- **Associated features** – Is it itchy? Is it sore or painful? Any discharge? Any burning or numbness? Does the rash disappear or go white if you press it?
- **Timing** – Is it always there? Has it changed? Have you had a similar rash before?
- **Exacerbating/relieving factors** – Can you think of anything that triggers it? Does anything make it better or worse? Are you using any new hand creams, perfumes, washing powders or other substances likely to contact the skin? Is it worse when you are in the sun?
- **Severity** – How is it affecting your day-to-day life?

SYSTEMS REVIEW

Note: These are screening questions; if a positive answer is given to any of them, it necessitates further probing about the symptom in question

- **Constitutional**–Have you been feeling unwell recently? Any fever, lethargy, loss of appetite or nausea?
- **RS** – Any recent infections? Recent cough?
- **GUT** – Any problems passing urine?
- **NS** – Any headache? Neck stiffness? Photophobia?
- **MSK** – Do you suffer from pain in your joints or your back? Painfully cold hands? Dry eyes or mouth? Ulcers? Hair loss?

RED FLAGS

Non-blanching rash
Headache
Neck stiffness
Photophobia
Generally unwell

PATIENT'S PERSPECTIVE

- **Feelings** – How do you feel about the rash from a psychological perspective?
- **Effect on life** – Has it affected your life in any way?
- **Ideas** – Do you have any idea yourself what might be causing the rash?

- **Concerns** – Is there anything you are particularly concerned about? Is there anything in general that concerns you about the rash?
- **Expectations** – Did you have anything particular in mind when you made the appointment to see me today?

BACKGROUND INFORMATION

PMH

- Do you suffer from any medical conditions or skin disorders?
- *Ask specifically about hay fever and asthma*

DH

- Are you currently taking any medications? Any herbal medicines or over-the-counter medicines?
- Have there been any changes to this in the last few months?
- Do you have any allergies to medications? Any other allergies?

FH

- Does anyone else in the family suffer with a similar condition?
- Do any conditions run in the family?
- *Ask specifically about hay fever and eczema*

SH

- Are you working presently? *If so,* what is your job? What does that involve? Do you come into contact with any harmful or irritating materials? Do you wear protection?
- Can you tell me about your home situation (*occupants and any difficulties*)?
- Has your rash caused any problems psychologically or otherwise at work or home?
- Does anyone else in the house have the same rash, or any other close contacts?
- Do you smoke? Do you drink alcohol?

CLOSING THE SESSION

- summary ± examination/explanation and planning/contract

IMPORTANT POINTS

- In an OSCE station, it is likely you will be asked to examine as well as take a history. Read the instructions carefully; you may only be allowed to ask a few pertinent questions rather than taking a full history
- Although examination of the rash is crucial in these OSCE stations, this should not be at the expense of a good *focused* history
- Some patients may walk in with visual clues (even simulated patients!) e.g. they may be wearing a hat to conceal their scalp psoriasis. If something appears different then comment on it and ask the patient about it – this will gain the interest of your examiner!
- Dermatological disorders can have a profound effect on the patient's psychological health, particularly in young females – be sure to ask how it is affecting them and about their concerns

DIFFERENTIAL DIAGNOSIS

ATOPIC ECZEMA (MOST COMMON)

- Suggested by a red exudative or scaly lesion, often with vesicles
- Usually on the flexor surfaces, face and neck, favouring skin creases
- Often very itchy – There may be evidence of excoriation or lichenification
- Family history of atopy such as asthma, hay fever or drug allergies

PURPURIC RASH (MOST SERIOUS)

- Small purple raised spots on the skin that do not blanch when pressed
- Wide range of causes, including meningococcal septicaemia (think red flags)
- Henoch–Schonlein purpura affects lower extremities and buttocks of children

PSORIASIS

- Typically, well-demarcated red scaly plaques (chronic plaque psoriasis), but pustular, guttate, erythrodermic and nail psoriatic varieties also exist
- Usually found on extensor surfaces
- Family history often present
- May be itchy; there may be an associated arthropathy and nail changes

CONTACT DERMATITIS

- Similar in presentation to eczema but with an irritant or allergic aetiology
- Commonly found on hands and may be linked to occupation e.g. a cleaner who reacts to soapy water

SEBORRHOEIC DERMATITIS

- A scaly, greasy, itchy rash that typically affects the scalp and face. Areas of the face affected include the nasolabial folds, eye brows and eyelids
- Dandruff is a common finding
- Can occur in newborns where it is known as cradle cap

VIRAL-INDUCED RASH

- The most common cause of a maculo-papular rash in children
- Usually a history of a preceding viral illness or malaise
- The rash blanches when pressed are not itchy or sore

VARICELLA ZOSTER

- Diffuse, itchy and painful vesicular and pustular lesions at different stages of development
- Shingles presents in immunocompromised adults in a dermatomal distribution
- Herpes zoster ophthalmicus may occur in trigeminal nerve involvement

URTICARIA

- White, itchy papule surrounded by erythema – multiple, localised or diffuse
- They occur very acutely, usually as a reaction to a topical allergen
- Can progress to anaphylaxis, which may result in angioedema
- Patients may have a history of hypersensitivity

CELLULITIS

- Well-demarcated erythematous rash, with swelling, warmth and tenderness
- Usually localised, often on the legs
- There may be tracking, whereby the rash spreads along the routes of the lymphatics
- Fever, tachycardia and malaise may be present

INVESTIGATIONS

- Full dermatological examination
- Dermoscopy for detailed examination of lesion
- Diascopy to reveal non-blanching rashes
- Biopsy to confirm diagnosis
- Skin scrapings for fungal infections
- Skin prick and patch testing
- Swabs if infection is suspected
- Wood's light can help highlight certain fungal infections such as tinea capitis
- FBC and clotting screen if purpuric rash
- Auto-antibody screen

MANAGEMENT

- A purpuric rash is managed based on its cause e.g. IV antibiotics for meningococcal septicaemia or splenectomy for treatment of recurrent idiopathic thrombocytopenic purpura
- **Seborrhoeic dermatitis** – Topical steroid cream for flare-ups and antifungal shampoo or cream for regular use to reduce relapses
- **Psoriasis** – Avoid excess drying of skin; encourage sun exposure; topical steroid and vitamin D analogue preparations; ultraviolet light/ PUVA therapy; coal tar; methotrexate or cyclosporin if these measures fail
- **Dermatitis** – Avoid precipitants, including soaps, creams and perfumes; topical moisturisers; topical steroids for flare-ups
- **Herpes zoster** – Oral aciclovir within 72 hours onset of rash
- **Cellulitis** – Oral antibiotics e.g. flucloxacillin

FURTHER READING

NICE CKS on:
Eczema, http://cks.nice.org.uk/eczema-atopic
Psoriasis, http://cks.nice.org.uk/psoriasis

BRUISING

INITIATING THE SESSION

- Greet the patient, ask an open question and screen for other problems

MEDICAL PERSPECTIVE

SEQUENCE OF EVENTS (SOCRATES)

- **Open question** – Can you tell me what has been going on? Start from the beginning
- **Site** – Where are the bruises? How many are there?
- **Onset** – When did you first notice the bruising? How has it progressed?
- **Character** – Can you describe the bruises? Are they large or like pin pricks?
- **Radiation** – Do you have any bruises elsewhere?
- **Associated features** – *See bleeding history*
- **Timing** – Have you been prone to bruising easily before?
- **Exacerbating/relieving factors** – Any recent bumps or injuries?
- **Severity** – Have you been feeling particularly ill or tired recently?

SYMPTOM ANALYSIS

- **Bleeding** – Do you tend to bleed very easily and for long periods when cut?
- **Menses** – Are your periods very heavy? Did you bleed much after giving birth?
- **Epistaxis** – Do you get nose bleeds frequently?
- **Rectal bleeding** – Is there ever any blood in your stools?
- **Haematuria** – Have you noticed any blood in your urine?
- **Post-op** – Have you ever had any trouble with massive bleeding after an operation?
- **Haemarthrosis** – Have you ever suffered with bleeding into the joints or muscle?

SYSTEMS REVIEW

- **Constitutional** – Have you recently been unwell with a flu-like illness? Do you feel more tired than normal? Have you noticed any weight loss? Have you noticed any lumps in your neck or elsewhere?
- **MSK** – Any aches and pains in your joints or muscles?
- **Infections** – Do you frequently get infections? Any infections recently?
- **Meningitis** – Have you had a headache? Neck stiffness? Sensitivity to light?

RED FLAGS

Fever
Meningitic features
Recurrent infections
Recent anaemia
Weight loss
Inconsistent history (kids)

PATIENT'S PERSPECTIVE

- **Feelings and effect on life** – How have your symptoms affected you?
- **Ideas** – Do you have any idea yourself what might be causing the bruising?
- **Concerns** – Is there anything you are particularly concerned about? Is there anything in general that concerns you about the bruising?
- **Expectations** – Did you have anything particular in mind when you made the appointment to see me today?

BACKGROUND INFORMATION

PMH

- Do you suffer from any medical conditions?
- *Ask specifically about blood disorders and previous malignancy*

DH

- What medications do you currently take? Do you take any over-the-counter medications?
- *Ask specifically about warfarin, aspirin, clopidogrel and newer anti-coagulants*
- Do you have any allergies?

FH

- Do any conditions run in your family?
- *Ask specifically about blood disorders*

SH

- Do you drink alcohol? How much do you drink in a week? How long has this been the case? *If required, take a more detailed alcohol history*
- Do you smoke? How many cigarettes do you smoke a day? For how long?
- Do you use any recreational drugs?
- Are you working presently? *If so,* what is your job? What does that involve?
- Can you tell me about your home situation (*occupants and any difficulties*)?
- Has your bruising affected your job or home life in any way?

CLOSING THE SESSION

- summary ± examination/explanation and planning/contract

IMPORTANT POINTS

- In children you *must* consider the possibility of non-accidental injury and safeguarding issues, including possibly interviewing the child alone. In adults, domestic abuse might still be a possibility. Truncal bruising is less likely to be due to accidental trauma
- Petechiae aren't necessarily pathological on the head/neck after vomiting
- In the drugs history, don't forget about over-the-counter and herbal remedies which can alter platelet function and coagulation factor levels. Pay particular attention to aspirin, steroids and warfarin. Also, has a warfarinised patient been taking antibiotics recently?
- A bleeding tendency can be the presenting feature of liver disease, so a good alcohol history is required

DIFFERENTIAL DIAGNOSIS

SIMPLE UNCOMPLICATED TRAUMA (MOST COMMON)

- Bruise preceded by an obvious trauma of appropriate force with local tenderness
- Common locations include the anterior aspect of lower legs and the forearms
- Less likely if the bruise is on the back, buttocks, upper arm or abdomen. It is also less likely benign if found in a child less than nine months old (less mobile)

NON-ACCIDENTAL INJURY (MOST SERIOUS)

- In the context of a paediatric history – history incompatible with child's developmental age; "old" bruises, limp, scald/burn marks suggest non-accidental injury
- Must involve paediatric consultant if suspicion arises, who will then involve social services – all part of a safeguarding team

HENOCH–SCHÖNLEIN PURPURA

- Typically affects younger children with a preceding URTI
- The rash looks very similar to bruises and starts on the back of the legs and buttocks or anywhere pressure is exerted such as sock tops. There may be associated abdominal pain, bloody diarrhoea, joint pain and in severe cases symptoms of renal failure

MONGOLIAN BLUE SPOT

- Birthmark frequently misdiagnosed as possible NAI
- Key is that mark has been present since birth

VITAMIN K DEFICIENCY

- In a newborn child, this should be considered
- It is possible that the child may not have been given vitamin K after birth
- In adults, due to liver disease or malabsorption with features of jaundice, history of alcohol abuse, steatorrhoea and weight loss

THROMBOCYTOPENIA

- Many causes including bone marrow failure, hypersplenism, haematological malignancy, uraemia and autoimmune disorders
- Poor platelet function often results in petechiae and mucosal bleeding
- Lymphadenopathy and recurrent infections may suggest leukaemia

HAEMOPHILIA A AND B

- Defects of factors VIII and IX, respectively; usually presents in childhood
- Hallmark symptoms of haemarthoses and muscle haematomas
- Severity depends on the level of functioning factor VIII/IX

VON WILLEBRAND'S DISEASE

- This is the most common inheritable bleeding tendency, affecting up to 1% of people. It is inherited in an autosomal dominant fashion
- Patients mainly complain of mucosal bleeding, although prolonged bleeding after surgery isn't uncommon

SENILE PURPURA

- Advanced age results in a decreased level of collagen, predisposing to bruising
- The bruises here are typically large and dark. The overlying skin is thin and fragile. These are usually found on extensor surfaces and forearms

COLLAGEN ABNORMALITY

- Abnormalities of the vessel walls and surrounding tissues can predispose to bleeding e.g. Ehlers–Danlos or Marfan's syndrome
- Skeletal involvement, cardiac involvement and ophthalmological involvement
- Features include hyper-extendable joints, tall stature and excess skin elasticity

INVESTIGATIONS

- FBC, LFTs, clotting and blood smear
- Bleeding time
- Mixing studies and factor + inhibitor assay
- Platelet antibody assay
- Bone marrow biopsy
- Urine analysis

MANAGEMENT

- **Haematological malignancy** – urgent referral to specialist services
- **NAI** – involvement of seniors and social services
- **HSP** – supportive treatment
- **Immune-thrombocytopenic purpura** is managed according to symptoms and monitored platelet levels; oral prednisolone or immunoglobulins in flare-ups; consider splenectomy in chronic relapsing cases
- **Haemophilia A and B** – recombinant factors VIII and IX, respectively
- **Vitamin K deficiency** – IM vitamin K injections

FURTHER READING

NICE CKS on bruising, http://cks.nice.org.uk/bruising

Cardiorespiratory medicine

CHEST PAIN

INITIATING THE SESSION

- Greet the patient, ask an open question and screen for other problems

MEDICAL PERSPECTIVE

SEQUENCE OF EVENTS

- **Open question** – Can you tell me more about this chest pain?
- **Timeline** – How did it come on? How did it progress from there?

SYMPTOM ANALYSIS (SOCRATES)

- **Site** – Where exactly is the pain? Can you point to where it is?
- **Onset** – When did it start? Did it come on suddenly or gradually? What were you doing at the time?
- **Character** – How would you describe the pain?
- **Radiation** – Does the pain go anywhere?
- **Associated factors** – *See systems review*
- **Timing** – Is the pain always there or does it come and go? What brings the pain on? Have you ever had this pain before?
- **Exacerbating/relieving factors** – Does anything make the pain better or worse? Is it worse when you walk? Does it go away with rest? Is there any relation to eating food? Is it better when you are in any particular position e.g. sitting up? Is it worse when taking deep breaths?
- **Severity** – How bad is the pain on a scale of 1–10, with 10 being the worst pain you can imagine? How would you score it at its worst?

SYSTEMS REVIEW

- **Dyspnoea** – Do you get breathless?
- **Orthopnoea** – Do you ever get breathless when lying flat? How many pillows do you sleep with at night?
- **Paroxysmal nocturnal dyspnoea** – Do you ever wake up gasping for breath?
- **Palpitations** – Do you ever get palpitations or an awareness of your heart beating? *If so*, are they fast, slow, regular or irregular?
- **Cough** – Have you noticed a cough? Do you bring anything up? Any blood?
- **Constitutional** – Have you noticed any weight loss? Do you feel sick with the pain? Has it made you sweat?
- **MSK** – Is the pain worse on movement? Does it hurt to press on the area?

PATIENT'S PERSPECTIVE

- **Feelings and effect on life** – How have your symptoms affected you?
- **Ideas** – Do you have any idea yourself what might be causing the pain?
- **Concerns** – Is there anything you are particularly concerned could be causing the pain? Is there anything in general that concerns you about the chest pain?
- **Expectations** – I understand the chest pain must be a worry. Would I be right in thinking you came today to check if it was something serious? Was there anything else you were hoping for?

BACKGROUND INFORMATION

PMH

- Do you suffer from any medical conditions?
- *Ask specifically about angina, diabetes, hypertension and reflux*
- **PE risk factors** – Do you have any clotting disorders? Have you ever had a cancer? Any recent surgery? Have you been on any long flights recently?

DH

- Do you take any regular medications, creams, sprays or pills? Any allergies?

FH

- Do any conditions run in the family? Is there any family history of heart disease? *If so, clarify the ages of onset in any immediate family members*
- *Ask specifically about hypercholesterolaemia and clotting disorders*

SH

- Do you smoke? (*Have you ever smoked/quantify*)
- Do you drink alcohol? How much do you drink in a week?
- Are you working presently? *If so,* what is your job? What does that involve? Has your problem affected your job in any way?
- Can you tell me about your home situation (*occupants and any difficulties*)? How is your problem affecting your home life?

CLOSING THE SESSION

- summary ± examination/explanation and planning/contract

IMPORTANT POINTS

- The patients most likely to appear in OSCEs are those with stable angina, a previous history of ACS, GORD or musculoskeletal pain
- The first important point to clarify is whether or not this is an acute event, as this may well push the working diagnosis more towards a more sinister cause
- Onset of heart disease in immediate family members before the age of 55 years in men and 65 years in women is considered a positive family history
- Cardiac pain is dull; often described as "tightness"/"discomfort"/"a heavy weight"
- "Sharp" pain is more likely parietal than visceral i.e. decreased probability of ACS
- Pleuritic pain (typically a sharp pain that is worse on breathing in) is less suggestive of IHD, and more of PE, pericarditis, pneumonia or costochondritis
- Dyspnoea, orthopnoea and paroxysmal nocturnal dyspnoea indicate heart failure

DIFFERENTIAL DIAGNOSIS

Think of cardiac causes in patients over the age of 50 years. Similarly, unless there is a family history, consider other causes in younger patients.

COMMON

STABLE ANGINA

- Central chest pain that may radiate to the arm and/or jaw
- Pain brought on by exercise and relieved by rest; no relation to food
- Associated breathlessness, but sweating, nausea and vomiting are not typical
- It is less likely to be simple angina if the pain remains after 20 minutes of rest and there is no relief from GTN spray

GASTRO-OESOPHAGEAL REFLUX DISEASE

- Retrosternal burning sensation, worse on lying flat, after eating large meals, bending forward or straining
- When describing the pain, the patient typically makes a fist and presses it up and down against his/her sternum
- Relieved by swallowing saliva, water or taking antacids
- Associated with the sensation of some regurgitation of acid and a sour taste

MUSCULOSKELETAL PAIN (INCLUDING COSTOCHONDRITIS AKA TIETZE'S SYNDROME)

- Localised, superficial pleuritic pain with no other associated symptoms
- There may or may not be a previous history of trauma
- Consider in younger patients with long-standing chest pain

PNEUMONIA

- History of cough and purulent sputum with general malaise and fever
- Pleuritic chest pain with haemoptysis, wheezing and shortness of breath.
- There may be a background history of respiratory disease (e.g. COPD)

SERIOUS

ACUTE CORONARY SYNDROME

- Sudden severe crushing central pain that may radiate to the arm and/or jaw
- Associated breathlessness, nausea, vomiting and sweating
- Typically, an old, obese male smoker with a sedentary lifestyle
- Angina often co-exists, but the pain is described as different to their usual pain

AORTIC DISSECTION

- Sudden onset of severe tearing/ripping pain felt between the shoulder blades
- Possible recent history of trauma including road traffic accidents; background of hypertension or Ehler–Danlos/Marfan's syndrome
- Wide range of secondary symptoms reflecting interruption of blood flow from the aorta, including acutely ischaemic limbs, stroke or even acute myocardial infarction

PULMONARY EMBOLISM

- Sudden onset of pleuritic pain; associated shortness of breath, fever and haemoptysis
- They may have noticed a swollen, hot tender leg unilaterally previously
- Risk factors include malignancy, pregnancy, clotting disorders, recent long-haul flights, or surgery with subsequent immobility

TENSION PNEUMOTHORAX

- Sudden onset of pleuritic chest pain with associated shortness of breath
- Background history of lung disease or collagen disease such as Marfan's syndrome or recent chest trauma (including recent insertion of a central line)

PERICARDITIS

- Pleuritic pain typically felt retrosternally and aggravated by coughing
- Classically the pain is better on sitting forward and worse on lying flat

INVESTIGATIONS

- Cardiorespiratory examination
- 12-lead ECG – perform promptly if ACS is suspected
- Bloods – FBC, U&Es, CRP and troponin (baseline and 12 hours); caution re D-dimer
- Chest x-ray
- CT angiogram if suspecting aortic dissection

- CTPA or V/Q scan if PE suspected
- Coronary angiography, functional imaging or CT calcium scoring for diagnosis of coronary artery disease (if stable angina suspected)
- Coronary angiography in ACS
- Endoscopy (urgent if red flags symptoms present, *see dysphagia history pp. 43*)

MANAGEMENT

- In suspected ACS, initially manage with morphine, high-flow oxygen, glyceryl trinitrate and aspirin (MONA) ± other antiplatelet and heparin as per local protocol; after confirmation of ACS, PCI or thrombolysis depending on services available locally; long-term management includes ACE inhibitors, beta-blockers and statins
- Aortic dissection – IV beta-blockers and nitrates initially; Stanford type A dissections require surgery; type B dissections are usually managed medically
- Tension pneumothorax – Large bore needle decompression in the second intercostal space mid-clavicular line, with subsequent chest drain placement, typically fifth intercostal space mid-axillary line
- PE – Low molecular weight heparin and warfarin commencement
- Reflux – Trial of protein pump inhibitor or test for *H. pylori* in first instance
- Angina – Beta-blocker or calcium channel antagonist is first-line therapy

FURTHER READING

NICE guidelines on assessment of chest pain, https://www.nice.org.uk/guidance/cg95

DYSPNOEA

INITIATING THE SESSION

- Greet the patient, ask an open question and screen for other problems

MEDICAL PERSPECTIVE

SEQUENCE OF EVENTS

- **Open question** – Can you tell me more about your breathlessness?
- **Clarify** – What exactly do you mean by breathlessness?
- **Timeline** – How did it start? How has it progressed since then?
- **Onset** – How long has this been going on for?

SYMPTOM ANALYSIS

- **Severity** – How far can you walk before the breathlessness stops you? Can you climb a flight of stairs in one go? *If not*, how many can you manage? Is it there at rest?
- **Relieving factors** – Does anything relieve your breathlessness when it comes on? If you rest for a while does it improve? Do inhalers help?
- **Exacerbating factors** – Does anything make it worse? Is it worse lying flat?
- **Orthopnoea/PND** – How many pillows do you sleep with? Do you have to prop yourself up? Do you ever wake up gasping for air?

SYSTEMS REVIEW

RED FLAGS

Chest pain
Haemoptysis
Weight loss
Heavy smoking history
Asbestos exposure
Unilateral leg swelling

- **Cough** – Have you noticed a cough? *If so*, for how long? Do you bring anything up? Have you noticed any blood?
- **Wheeze** – Do you get wheezy? Is it worse at any time of the day?
- **Chest pain** – Do you suffer from chest pain? *If so, SOCRATES*
- **Palpitations** – Do you get palpitations along with the breathlessness? *If so*, are they fast, slow, regular or irregular?
- **PE** – Have you noticed any leg swelling? Any recent long distance travel/surgery/immobility?
- **Constitutional** – Have you felt hot and cold or feverish? Have you had any weight loss? How is your appetite?
- **Psychiatric** – *If relevant*, do you only get breathless when you are anxious?

PATIENT'S PERSPECTIVE

- **Feelings and effect on life** – How have your symptoms affected your daily life?
- **Ideas** – Do you have any ideas what might be causing the difficulty in breathing?
- **Concerns** – Is there anything you are particularly concerned could be causing it? Is there anything in general that concerns you about the breathlessness?
- **Expectations** – Was there anything in particular you were hoping for when you made the appointment for today?

BACKGROUND INFORMATION

PMH

- Do you suffer from any medical conditions?
- *Ask specifically about asthma, COPD and heart disease*

DH

- Are you currently taking any medication? Do you have any allergies?
- Do you have oxygen at home? Do you use nebulisers?

FH

- Do any conditions run in the family?
- *Ask specifically about ischaemic heart disease and asthma*

SH

- Do you smoke? How many cigarettes do you smoke a day? For how long?
- What is/was your job? *If relevant,* did that involve working with asbestos?
- How are you managing at home? Do you have stairs?

CLOSING THE SESSION

- summary ± examination/explanation and planning/contract

> **IMPORTANT POINTS**
>
> - Try to quantify their breathlessness. Sedentary patients complaining of being breathless on walking to their bathroom may be more significant than an aging athlete who can't complete a marathon anymore
> - As a general rule, if a patient can climb the stairs in one go, they should be capable of having a lung removed without significant impairment
> - COPD is less likely if there is less than a 20 pack-year history
> - You need to assess to what extent the patients' dyspnoea affects their life. There may not be a need for aggressive intervention if their symptoms are not intrusive

DIFFERENTIAL DIAGNOSIS

ACUTE/SUB-ACUTE

Asthma exacerbation

- Sudden onset of wheezing and breathlessness
- Often precipitated by a trigger such as exercise, cold air, dust or pollen
- Recurrent problem, often with atopic background (e.g. eczema and hay fever)
- Diurnal variation of asthma classically causes night-time coughing

Pneumonia

- History of cough and purulent sputum with general malaise and fever
- Pleuritic chest pain with haemoptysis, wheezing and shortness of breath
- There may be a background history of respiratory disease (e.g. COPD)

Acute pulmonary oedema

- Severe breathlessness often precipitated by ACS, arrhythmia or deterioration of deteriorating renal function
- Orthopnoea, paroxysmal nocturnal dyspnoea and cough (frothy pink sputum)

Acute coronary syndrome

- Sudden, severe, crushing central pain that may radiate to the arm and/or jaw
- May be "silent" though, with only breathlessness, particularly in the elderly
- Associated nausea, vomiting and sweating

Pulmonary embolism

- Sudden onset of pleuritic pain with breathlessness, fever and haemoptysis
- There may have been a swollen, hot tender leg unilaterally previously
- Risk factors include malignancy, pregnancy, clotting disorders, recent long-haul flights or surgery with subsequent immobility

Tension pneumothorax

- Sudden onset of pleuritic chest pain with associated shortness of breath
- Background history of lung disease or collagen disease such as Marfan's syndrome or recent chest trauma (including recent insertion of a central line)

CHRONIC

Lung malignancy

- Weight loss and haemoptysis are red flags; significant smoking history
- Progressive breathlessness, hoarse voice, dysphagia, wheezing, stridor, recurrent chest infections and chest discomfort are all features
- Paraneoplastic syndrome also possible due to ectopic hormone production e.g. Cushing's or syndrome of inappropriate antidiuretic hormone secretion (SIADH) – These are usually related to small cell lung cancer

Chronic obstructive pulmonary disease

- Constant breathlessness, long smoking history, chronic cough, wheeze and sputum
- Progressive with increasing exertional dyspnoea and increasing disability
- Can also develop acute, infective and non-infective exacerbations that can present similarly to an asthma exacerbation

Interstitial lung disease

- Chronic and progressive breathlessness on exertion
- Wheezing, chest pain, haemoptysis and sputum are not typically seen
- Many environmental and occupational risk factors e.g. farmer's lung

Chronic heart failure

- Exertional dyspnoea, orthopnoea and paroxysmal nocturnal dyspnoea
- Background history of heart disease (e.g. IHD or hypertension)

INVESTIGATIONS

- Full cardiorespiratory examination and bedside observations
- ECG
- FBC, U&Es, cardiac markers and BNP
- ABG
- Chest x-ray
- Peak flow and pulmonary function tests for asthma and COPD, respectively
- CTPA or V/Q scan to look for PE
- Echocardiography to assess heart failure
- Coronary angiogram to assess for acute coronary syndrome
- High-resolution CT of chest to assess for pulmonary fibrosis

MANAGEMENT

- ABCDE approach in acutely unwell patients if unable to give history
- Smoking cessation and pulmonary rehabilitation are key in the long term
- Oxygen should be given to any patient with low saturations, with target range of 94–98% in most patients, and 88–92% in those with COPD
- Acute exacerbation – 100% oxygen, inhaled or nebulised salbutamol and oral/IV steroids; ipratropium, magnesium sulphate and ICU referral if poor response
- In suspected ACS, initially manage with morphine, 100% oxygen, nitrate (GTN spray) and aspirin (MONA); after confirmation of ACS, PCI or thrombolysis depending on services available locally; long-term management includes ACE inhibitors, beta-blockers and statins
- Acute pulmonary oedema – IV furosemide and nitrate infusion as BP tolerates
- COPD exacerbation – Antibiotics, bronchodilators, oxygen and steroids
- PE – Low molecular weight heparin and warfarin commencement
- Pneumonia – Antibiotics; a CURB 65 score of 2 or more requires admission

FURTHER READING

NICE CKS on breathlessness, http://cks.nice.org.uk/breathlessness

PALPITATIONS

INITIATING THE SESSION

- Greet the patient, ask an open question and screen for other problems

MEDICAL PERSPECTIVE

SEQUENCE OF EVENTS

- **Open question** – Can you tell me more about these palpitations?
- **Timeline** – How did you first notice them? How have things progressed since then?

SYMPTOM ANALYSIS (SOCRATES)

- **Specify** – What exactly do you mean by palpitations?
- **Onset** – When did you first notice them?
- **Character** – When they occur, does your heart pound fast or slow?
- **Rhythm** – Do they feel regular or irregular?
- **Associated features** – *See systems review*
- **Timing** – How long do they last for? Do they come on at a particular time? During exercise? How often do you get palpitations?
- **Exacerbating/relieving factors** – Does anything help stop the palpitations?
- **Severity** – How do you feel when these palpitations come on?

SYSTEMS REVIEW

<table>
<tr><td>

RED FLAGS

Associated with exertion
Chest pain
Collapse
Family history of sudden unexpected death

</td></tr>
</table>

- **CVS** – Do you get any chest pain with the palpitations? Breathlessness? Dizzy spells or faints?
- **Psychiatric** – Do the attacks typically follow episodes of anxiety or panic?
- **Endocrine** – Do you find yourself feeling hot all the time? Have you lost weight recently? Do you get diarrhoea? Are your periods regular? When your palpitations occur, do you also get sweaty and nauseous? Do you have high blood pressure?

PATIENT'S PERSPECTIVE

- **Feelings and effect on life** – How have the palpitations affected you?
- **Ideas** – Do you have any ideas what might be causing the palpitations?
- **Concerns** – Is there anything you are particularly concerned could be causing it? Is there anything in general that concerns you about them?
- **Expectations** – Was there anything in particular you were hoping for when you made the appointment for today?

BACKGROUND INFORMATION

PMH

- Do you suffer from any medical conditions?
- *Ask specifically about heart disease, psychiatric history and thyroid disorders*

DH

- Are you currently taking any medications? Do you have any allergies?

FH

- Do any conditions run in the family?
- *Ask specifically about heart disease and sudden unexpected deaths*

SH

- Do you smoke? Do you drink alcohol? Do you take any recreational drugs?
- Do you drink much tea, coffee or other caffeinated drinks?
- Are you working presently? *If so,* what is your job? What does that involve?
- Can you tell me about your home situation (*occupants and any difficulties*)?
- Has your problem affected your job or home life in any way?

CLOSING THE SESSION

- summary ± examination/explanation and planning/contract

IMPORTANT POINTS

- Identifying patients with a propensity to sudden cardiac death is certainly one of the main objectives in assessing palpitation patients
- A family history of sudden cardiac death is very significant and warrants a more urgent investigation
- Palpitations brought on by minimal exercise/stress can be a sign of significant cardiac pathology

DIFFERENTIAL DIAGNOSIS

CARDIAC CAUSES

Palpitations may represent an arrhythmia, but most arrhythmias do not produce palpitations. Syncope or a history of IHD makes ventricular tachycardia and other serious arrhythmias more likely, requiring more prompt investigation.

Ventricular tachycardia (most serious)

- Often short lived and asymptomatic, but prolonged episodes may cause haemodynamic compromise
- Typically occurs in patients with cardiac pathology such as IHD, heart failure, cardiomyopathies or long QT syndrome
- Family history may reveal a sudden death in a family member

Atrial fibrillation

- Often asymptomatic but there may be signs and symptoms of heart failure
- There may be a recent history of a cardiac event or major surgery

- May be paroxysmal, persistent or permanent
- Causes include IHD, valvular disease, thyrotoxicosis, alcohol and pneumonia

Supraventricular tachycardia

- Paroxysmal palpitations and sometimes associated syncope
- E.g. Wolff–Parkinson–White syndrome

Ectopic beats

- Typically, patients feel a skipped beat, followed by an uncomfortable lurch in the chest; some patients describe an inability to catch their breath
- The palpitations may be more evident when the patient lies flat, commonly at night time (related to the natural slowing of the heart rate at this time)

NON-CARDIAC CAUSES

Anxiety (most common)

- History of anxiety, agitations, sweating, nausea and dry mouth
- An intense feeling of panic or anxiety usually precedes the palpitations
- Palpitations are often regular, slightly fast and tend to come and go gradually

Thyrotoxicosis

- History of weight loss, heat intolerance, hair loss, altered appetite, loose bowels, tremor, neck swelling, palpitations and menstrual irregularity

Phaeochromocytoma

- Very rare catecholamine-secreting tumour of the adrenal glands
- Patient typically presents with hypertension, sweats, palpitations and tremor
- May be associated with multiple endocrine neoplasia type 2 (medullary thyroid carcinoma, parathyroid gland hyperplasia and phaeochromocytoma)

INVESTIGATIONS

- Full cardiovascular examination
- 12-lead ECG
- 24–48 hour ambulatory ECG tape
- Transtelephonic event monitoring for less frequent attacks
- FBC, U&Es and TFTs
- Urgent echocardiogram if any red flags are present/concern about cardiomyopathy
- Anxiety questionnaire e.g. HAD10
- Electrophysiological studies
- BP monitoring and 24-hour urine catecholamines if suspecting phaeochromocytoma

MANAGEMENT

- Avoid substances that predispose to palpitations, such as caffeine and alcohol
- Supraventricular tachycardias – vagal manoeuvres (e.g. carotid massage or valsalva manoeuvre); IV adenosine if vagal manoeuvres fail; radiofrequency catheter ablation of an identified focus for long-term cure

- Ventricular tachycardia – High-flow oxygen; if haemodynamically unstable, treat as a cardiac arrest according to ALS protocol; if stable, may initially be treated with lignocaine or amiodarone; if there is underlying structural heart disease, prophylactic medication and an implantable cardio-defibrillator should be considered
- Thyrotoxicosis – Propranolol; carbimazole/propylthiouracil; Radioiodine or subtotal/total thyroidectomy (plus lifelong thyroxine) if anti-thyroid drugs fail
- Atrial fibrillation – Rate control achieved using either beta-blockers or rate-limiting calcium channel blockers; rhythm control achieved using flecainide, IV amiodarone or by DC cardioversion; if high risk of stroke, start warfarin
- Anxiety – Counselling, CBT, SSRIs or benzodiazepines for severe anxiety; symptoms can be controlled with beta-blockers
- Ectopic beats – Usually no treatment required; they are not associated with a poor prognosis, and education is all that is needed to reassure patients

FURTHER READING

NICE CKS summary on palpitations, http://cks.nice.org.uk/palpitations

COUGH

INITIATING THE SESSION

- Greet the patient, ask an open question and screen for other problems

MEDICAL PERSPECTIVE

SEQUENCE OF EVENTS

- **Open question** – Can you tell me more about the cough?
- **Timeline** – When did you first notice the cough? Has it changed recently?
- **Timing** – Is it there all the time? Is it worse at any particular time of the day? Does it vary with the seasons or weather?
- **Triggers** – Does anything set the cough off?

SYMPTOM ANALYSIS

- **Sputum** – Do you cough anything up or is it a dry cough? *If so,* how much? What colour is it? Do you normally cough anything up?
- **Blood** – Do you ever cough up blood? Is it mixed in or streaky? How long has this been going on for?

RED FLAGS

Haemoptysis/brown sputum
Weight loss
Cough present >3 weeks
Chest pain
Foreign travel

SYSTEMS REVIEW

- **Wheeze** – Have you noticed a wheeze or any other strange sounds?
- **Dyspnoea** – Have you been breathless? *If so, quantify exercise tolerance*
- **Chest pain** – Do you have any chest pain?
- **URTI** – Do you have a cold? Is your nose runny or blocked or your throat sore?
- **GIT** – Do you suffer from heartburn? Is your cough worse on lying flat?
- **Constitutional** – Have you been feeling generally unwell with fever and chills? Have you recently lost any weight? How is your appetite?

PATIENT'S PERSPECTIVE

- **Feelings and effect on life** – How has the cough affected you?
- **Ideas** – Do you have any ideas yourself about what could be causing the cough?
- **Concerns** – Is there anything you are particularly concerned could be causing it? Is there anything in general that concerns you about your cough?
- **Expectations** – Was there anything in particular you were hoping for when you made the appointment for today?

BACKGROUND INFORMATION

PMH

- Do you suffer from any medical conditions?
- *Ask specifically about asthma and COPD*

DH

- Are you currently taking any medications? Do you have any allergies?
- *Ask specifically about ACE inhibitors*

FH

- Do any conditions run in the family?
- *Ask specifically about asthma*

SH

- Have you travelled anywhere abroad in the last 6 months?
- Do you smoke? How many cigarettes do you smoke a day? For how long?
- Are you working presently? *If so,* what is your job? What does that involve? Has there been any exposure to asbestos?
- Can you tell me about your home situation (*occupants and any difficulties*)?
- Has your problem affected your job or home life in any way?

CLOSING THE SESSION

- summary ± examination/explanation and planning/contract

IMPORTANT POINTS

- The occupational history is very important for a chronic cough – Legal proceedings against employers are very common now especially for conditions such as asbestosis, for which a properly documented cough history and exposure to harmful substances is vital
- In a child, consider the possibility of an inhaled foreign body, especially where there is a prominent stridor

DIFFERENTIAL DIAGNOSIS

ACUTE (<3 WEEKS)

URTI/post-nasal drip (most common)

- This is a common cause of a cough in a non-smoking adult
- Short history of an irritating cough with a recent URTI, but otherwise well
- Runny nose, congestion, sore throat, sinusitis and throat clearing

Pneumonia

- History of cough and purulent sputum production with malaise and fever
- There may be pleuritic chest pain, haemoptysis, wheezing and breathlessness
- Often a background history of respiratory disease (e.g. COPD/bronchiectasis)

ACE inhibitors

- ACE inhibitors cause a dry cough in 5 to 20% of patients
- No other symptoms present
- Usually presents within a week of starting therapy, but can be up to 6 months

SUB-ACUTE (3–8 WEEKS)

Lung malignancy (most serious)

- Weight loss and haemoptysis are red flags; significant smoking history
- Progressive breathlessness, hoarse voice, dysphagia, wheezing, stridor, recurrent chest infections and chest discomfort are all features
- Paraneoplastic syndrome also possible due to ectopic hormone production e.g. Cushing's syndrome or SIADH – These are usually related to small cell lung cancer

Gastro-oesophageal reflux disease

- Typically, overweight patient with retrosternal burning pain worse on lying flat
- Acid brash, with regurgitation of sour material after eating large meals
- May have a hoarse voice in the morning and periodically clear their throat

CHRONIC (>8 WEEKS)

Asthma

- Diurnal variation – Cough worse at night and in the morning
- Coughing is worse in cold air or after exercise
- May be associated with wheezing and breathlessness
- Often a background history of atopy, such as eczema and hay fever

Chronic obstructive pulmonary disease

- Constant breathlessness, with episodes of exacerbation due to infection
- Long smoking history, with chronic cough, wheeze and sputum production
- Progressive, with increasing exertional dyspnoea and increasing disability

Bronchiectasis

- Precipitated by recurrent infections or a particularly bad chest infection
- Production of large amounts of sputum ("cupfuls") each day
- Haemoptysis and breathlessness may be present
- Cystic fibrosis is associated with bronchiectasis

INVESTIGATIONS

- Full cardiorespiratory examination
- FBC, U&Es, LFTs and blood culture
- Sputum culture
- Chest x-ray
- Peak flow and pulmonary function tests for asthma and COPD, respectively
- CT thorax
- Bronchoscopy

MANAGEMENT

- Pneumonia – Antibiotics; a CURB 65 score of 2 or more requires admission
- Asthma – Stepwise approach, starting with inhaled salbutamol PRN; regular inhaled corticosteroid may be added, and then a long acting beta2-agonist; leukotriene antagonists, theophylline and oral steroids may also be needed

- COPD – Stop smoking, inhaled bronchodilators, inhaled corticosteroids and consider long-term domiciliary oxygen therapy
- Lung cancer – Urgent referral; surgery, chemotherapy and/or radiotherapy
- Reflux – Proton pump inhibitor and antacids
- ACE inhibitor cough – Stop and switch to angiotensin receptor blocker

FURTHER READING

NICE CKS on cough, http://cks.nice.org.uk/cough

NICE guidelines on lung cancer, https://www.nice.org.uk/guidance/ng12/chapter/
  1-Recommendations-organised-by-site-of-cancer#lung-and-pleural-cancers

HAEMOPTYSIS

INITIATING THE SESSION

- Greet the patient, ask an open question and screen for other problems

MEDICAL PERSPECTIVE

SEQUENCE OF EVENTS AND SYMPTOM ANALYSIS

- **Open question** – Can you tell me exactly what you have noticed?
- **Site** – Can I just check you are coughing up blood, not vomiting it up? Any recent nose bleeds?
- **Timeline** – When did you first notice it? How many times have you noticed it?
- **Colour** – What colour is it? *Bright red or dark brown*
- **Amount** – How much are you coughing up? Streaks or larger amounts?

SYSTEMS REVIEW

- **Cough** – Have you been coughing before you recently noticed the blood? *If so,* how long have you had a cough for? Is it there all the time?
- **Sputum** – Do you cough up sputum? *If so,* what colour is it? How much do you bring up? Streaks or cupfuls?
- **Chest pain** – Do you have chest pain? *If so, SOCRATES*
- **Dyspnoea** – Are you short of breath? *If so, quantify exercise tolerance.* Do your ankles swell?
- **Constitutional** – Any recent weight loss? How is your appetite? Have you been feeling feverish? Any night sweats? *If so,* are they drenching? Have you noticed any lumps or enlarged glands?
- **PE** – Any long-haul flights recently? Recent surgery? Swollen legs? Have you suffered from blood clots in the past?
- **Travel** – Have you travelled anywhere outside the UK within the last year?

PATIENT'S PERSPECTIVE

- **Feelings and effect on life** – I understand that this can be frightening. How has it affected you?
- **Ideas** – Do you have any ideas yourself about what could be causing your symptoms?
- **Concerns** – Is there anything you are particularly concerned could be causing it? Is there anything in general that concerns you?
- **Expectations** – Would I be right in thinking that you have come in today mainly to try to find out what is causing it? Was there anything else you were hoping for today?

BACKGROUND INFORMATION

PMH

- Do you suffer from any medical conditions?
- *Ask specifically about cancer, bleeding and clotting disorders*

DH

- Are you currently taking any medications? Do you have any allergies?
- *Ask specifically about warfarin and the combined oral contraceptive pill*

FH

- Do any conditions run in your family?
- *Ask specifically about clotting disorders and bleeding disorders*

SH

- Do you smoke? How many cigarettes do you smoke a day? For how long?
- Do you drink alcohol? How much do you drink in a week?
- Are you working presently? *If so,* what is your job? What does that involve?
- Can you tell me about your home situation (*occupants and any difficulties*)?
- Has your problem affected your job or home life in any way?

CLOSING THE SESSION

- summary ± examination/explanation and planning/contract

> **IMPORTANT POINTS**
>
> - Be sure to get an accurate smoking history in anyone with haemoptysis to properly assess their risk for lung cancer – if they say they don't smoke, ask if they have ever smoked and determine their pack-year history
> - It can be hard to distinguish true haemoptysis from other sources, so clarify with them that they are definitely coughing it up and ask about non-pulmonary causes such as nose bleeds or poor dental hygiene
> - It is important to ask about risk factors for PE to rule it out in cases of haemoptysis

DIFFERENTIAL DIAGNOSIS

ACUTE BRONCHITIS (MOST COMMON)

- Few day's history of fever, malaise and cough with shortness of breath
- Mucopurulent sputum streaked with blood

LUNG MALIGNANCY (MOST SERIOUS)

- Weight loss and haemoptysis are red flags for lung cancer
- Patients may also complain of progressive breathlessness, a hoarse voice, dysphagia, wheezing or stridor, recurrent chest infections or chest discomfort
- Risk factors include increasing age, smoking history, occupational exposure to asbestos and other hazardous industrial dusts
- Patients may also have symptoms of a paraneoplastic syndrome such as Cushing's (central obesity, bruising, thin skin etc.), dermatomyositis or SIADH

PULMONARY EMBOLISM

- Pleuritic chest pain with shortness of breath
- Associated fever, tachycardia and occasionally haemoptysis
- Possible background history of a pro-coagulant state such as malignancy, pregnancy or anti-thrombin 3 deficiency
- Similarly, there may be a history of recent air travel or operation with long periods of immobilisation. The patient may also complain of a painful swollen leg

PNEUMONIA

- Rapid onset over a day or so of shortness of breath, cough, pleuritic chest pain, fever and general malaise
- Classically rusty brown sputum

TUBERCULOSIS

- Long-standing fever, malaise, lymphadenopathy and weight loss
- Classically produces night sweats
- Risk factors for infection including immunosuppression, travel to endemic areas, alcoholism and IV drug users

LUNG ABSCESS

- Production of copious amounts of blood-stained foul-smelling sputum
- Often significant preceding pneumonia or similar seeding event such as infective endocarditis, foreign body aspiration or trauma
- Swinging fevers, pleuritic chest pain, cough and weight loss

BRONCHIECTASIS

- Precipitated by recurrent infections or a particularly bad chest infection
- Production of large amounts of sputum ("cupfuls") each day
- Haemoptysis and breathlessness may be present
- Cystic fibrosis is associated with bronchiectasis

INVESTIGATIONS

- Look at the sputum. Is there any blood? Send sputum culture
- FBC, U&Es, LFTs, clotting, CRP and ESR
- D-dimer may be considered to rule out PE $\pm$ CTPA
- Blood cultures
- Mantoux test/Quantiferon-TB Gold
- Chest x-ray
- CT chest
- Bronchoscopy

MANAGEMENT

- PE – High-dose low-molecular-weight heparin and warfarin
- Tuberculosis – 6 months treatment with isoniazid and rifampicin with the addition for the first 2 months of pyrazinamide and ethambutol
- Pneumonia – Antibiotics; a CURB 65 score of 2 or more requires admission
- Lung cancer – Urgent referral; surgery, chemotherapy and/or radiotherapy
- Bronchiectasis – Antibiotics; mucolytics and chest physiotherapy; bronchial artery embolization can be considered for massive haemoptysis
- Lung abscess – IV antibiotics; percutaneous drainage via CT guidance

FURTHER READING

NICE guidelines on tuberculosis, https://www.nice.org.uk/guidance/ng33

Gastroenterology

DYSPHAGIA

INITIATING THE SESSION

- Greet the patient, ask an open question and screen for other problems

MEDICAL PERSPECTIVE

SEQUENCE OF EVENTS

- **Open question** – Can you tell me more about your difficulty swallowing?
- **Timeline** – How did it start? How long ago? How has it progressed since then?
- **Timing** – Is it there all the time or does it come and go?

SYMPTOM ANALYSIS

- **Solids or liquids?** – Do you have difficulty swallowing solids, fluids or both?
- **Nature of dysphagia** – Does food get stuck in your throat when swallowing? Do you ever feel a lump in your throat? Have you noticed having bad-smelling breath? Do you ever notice gurgling or a wet voice after swallowing?

SYSTEMS REVIEW

- **GORD** – Do you suffer from reflux or indigestion?
- **Haematemesis** – Have you vomited at all? *If so,* was there any blood?
- **Bowel habit** – Have you noticed any change in your bowels? How many times a day do you go to the toilet? Has that changed at all? Have you noticed any blood in your stools? Is it darker or more smelly than usual?
- **NS** – Have you noticed any weakness anywhere? Any problems walking? Any change in your vision or other senses?

RED FLAGS

Progressive dysphagia
Anaemia (unexplained)
Weight loss
Anorexia
Melaena/haematemesis
Age >55 years

- **MSK** – Do you suffer with painfully cold hands that change colour? Dry eyes or mouth? Tight, shiny skin? Have you noticed any change in your appearance?
- **Constitutional** – Have you had any weight loss? *If so,* how much have you lost and over how long?

PATIENT'S PERSPECTIVE

- **Feelings and effect on life** – How have your symptoms affected you?
- **Ideas** – Do you have any ideas yourself about what could be going on?
- **Concerns** – Is there anything you are particularly concerned could be causing it? Is there anything in general that concerns you?
- **Expectations** – I understand this can be a scary problem. Was there anything in particular you had in mind that you were hoping for today?

BACKGROUND INFORMATION

PMH

- Do you suffer from any medical conditions?
- *Ask specifically about neurological conditions such as multiple sclerosis and previous history of stroke and/or malignancy*
- Have you ever, accidentally or otherwise, drunk corrosives such as bleach?

DH

- Do you take any medications? Any over-the-counter medications? Any allergies?
- *Ask specifically about NSAIDs and steroids*

FH

- Do any conditions run in the family?

SH

- Do you smoke? How many do you smoke/day? For how many years?
- Do you drink alcohol? How much do you drink in a week?
- Are you working presently? *If so,* what is your job? What does that involve?
- Can you tell me about your home situation (*occupants and any difficulties*)?
- Has your problem affected your job or home life in any way?

CLOSING THE SESSION

- summary ± examination/explanation and planning/contract

IMPORTANT POINTS

- Dysphagia is a red flag for sinister pathology and warrants a 2-week wait referral
- Make sure you cover all of the red flags (*see red flags box*)
- It is good to get an idea straight away about how long the problem has been going on and how things are progressing – if the nature hasn't changed and it has been there for years, sinister causes are less likely
- Untreated dysphagia can lead to malnutrition, pneumonia and even aspiration

DIFFERENTIAL DIAGNOSIS

NEUROMUSCULAR DISORDERS

Stroke

- Other features include acute onset of speech impairment and limb weakness
- High risk of aspiration, with gurgling voice after drinking
- Risk factors include diabetes, obesity, hypertension and atrial fibrillation

Myasthenia gravis

- Autoimmune neuromuscular disorder characterised by muscle fatigability
- Difficulty initiating swallowing and subsequent coughing due to aspiration
- Other signs and symptoms include weakness, ptosis, dysarthria, shortness of breath and waddling gait

Motor neurone disease

- Age is usually between 50 and 70 years and more commonly seen in males
- Progressive illness associated with upper and lower motor signs
- In progressive bulbar palsy, quiet hoarse voice and difficulties swallowing may be the first presenting symptoms

OBSTRUCTIVE DISORDERS

Oesophageal cancer (most severe)

- Progressively worsening dysphagia, initially for solids but later also for liquids
- The red flag symptoms suggest possibility and necessitate urgent referral
- Risk factors include advanced age, male sex, smoking, high alcohol intake and chronic GORD (Barrett's oesophagus)

Benign oesophageal stricture

- Associated with chronic GORD (acid brash and retrosternal burning pain)
- Intermittent dysphagia for solids which gradually worsens over time
- There may be a history of corrosive ingestion, radiation exposure or trauma

Oesophageal web

- Associated with odynophagia
- Either due to congenital defect or Plummer–Vinson syndrome
- Plummer–Vinson syndrome – chronic iron-deficiency anaemia with web

Pharyngeal pouch

- Sensation of lump in throat and halitosis

External oesophageal compression

- Retrosternal goitre or other mediastinal masses such as lymphomas

OESOPHAGEAL MOTILITY DISORDERS

Achalasia

- Impaired relaxation of lower oesophageal sphincter
- Long history of intermittent dysphagia for solids more than liquids
- Retrosternal chest pain after meals and heartburn are associated features

Oesophageal spasm

- Spontaneous intermittent chest pain commonly misdiagnosed as ACS

Systemic sclerosis

- Reflux symptoms as well as tight, thickened skin causing characteristic appearance, Raynaud's phenomenon and possible lung/heart involvement

OTHERS

- Globus pharyngeus – Somatisation disorder with sensation of lump in throat; anxiety may co-exist
- Tonsillitis – Difficulty swallowing here is due to pain

INVESTIGATIONS

- Full neck and abdominal examination
- Bloods – FBC, U&Es, LFTs and clotting and bone profile
- Chest x-ray
- Barium swallow
- Endoscopy and biopsy
- Videofluoroscopy – assessing for aspiration
- Staging CT scan, depending on what the previous investigations reveal

MANAGEMENT

- 2-week referral for patients with red flag symptoms
- Dietician referral for further input and assessment of nutrition
- Speech and language therapy to assess safety of swallow (risk of aspiration)
- Benign stricture – Slow meals and quantity, antacids and endoscopic dilatation
- Achalasia – Smooth muscle dilator and endoscopic dilatation
- Calcium channel blocker in oesophageal spasm
- Systemic sclerosis – Small meals and rheumatology referral
- Psychological therapy may be of assistance to patients with globus pharyngeus

FURTHER READING

NICE CKS on upper GI cancer recognition, http://cks.nice.org.uk/gastrointestinal-tract-upper-cancers-recognition-and-referral

HAEMATEMESIS

INITIATING THE SESSION

- Greet the patient, ask an open question and screen for other problems

MEDICAL PERSPECTIVE

SEQUENCE OF EVENTS

- **Open question** – Can you tell me more about what has been going on?
- **Timeline** – When did this start? How has it progressed?
- **Timing** – Has this happened before? *If so,* what happened then?

SYMPTOM ANALYSIS

- **Clarify site** – Is the blood definitely in your vomit, and not from coughing or a nosebleed? Is it fresh red blood or coffee ground colour?
- **Amount** – How much blood have you noticed? Streaks? A teaspoon? More?
- **Trigger** – Did anything trigger the bleeding? Were you retching before vomiting up blood?

SYSTEMS REVIEW

- **GORD** – Have you been suffering from indigestion or reflux? Any abdominal pain?
- **Bowel habit/melaena** – Have you noticed any change in your bowels? How many times a day do you go to the toilet? Have you noticed any blood in your stools? Is it darker or more smelly than usual?
- **Dysphagia** – Have you had any difficulty swallowing?
- **Constitutional** – How have your energy levels been recently? Have you had any recent unintentional weight loss? *If so,* how much have you lost and over how long? How has your appetite been?
- **Hepatic** – Have you noticed a yellow tinge to your skin? Is your skin itchy? Has your abdomen become more swollen or felt bloated?

> **RED FLAGS**
>
> Dysphagia
> Anaemia (unexplained)
> Weight loss
> Anorexia
> Age >55 years
> Jaundice

PATIENT'S PERSPECTIVE

- **Feelings and effect on life** – How have your symptoms affected you?
- **Ideas** – Do you have any ideas yourself about what could be going on?
- **Concerns** – Is there anything you are particularly concerned could be causing it? Is there anything in general that concerns you?
- **Expectations** – I understand this can be a scary problem. Was there anything in particular you had in your mind that you were hoping for today?

BACKGROUND INFORMATION

PMH

- Do you suffer from any medical conditions?
- *Ask specifically about liver disease, peptic ulcers, previous malignancy and surgery*

DH

- Do you take any regular medications? Any over-the-counter medications?
- *Ask specifically about NSAIDs, anti-platelets, anti-coagulants and steroids*

FH

- Do any conditions run in the family?
- *Ask specifically about malignancy (gastric carcinoma) and bleeding disorders*

SH

- Do you smoke? How many cigarettes do you smoke a day? How long have you smoked for?
- Do you drink alcohol? How much do you drink in a week?
- Do you take any recreational drugs? *If so,* do you inject any drugs?
- Are you working presently? *If so,* what is your job? What does that involve?
- Can you tell me about your home situation (*occupants and any difficulties*)?
- Has your problem affected your job or home life in any way?

CLOSING THE SESSION

- summary ± examination/explanation and planning/contract

IMPORTANT POINTS

- Gauge from the start whether the patient is acutely unwell or if they are comfortable and able to talk after a previous episode – this will determine whether you should proceed with a full history or whether you should start a more appropriate acute management approach (i.e. ABCDE)
- It is important to distinguish haematemesis from haemoptysis or a nosebleed
- Don't forget to ask about the red flag symptoms
- The colour and amount of vomitus can be used to guide potential severity and origin – coffee ground vomit suggests a bleed that has been exposed to gastric acid, whereas a large amount of fresh red bleeding may suggest a large haemorrhage

DIFFERENTIAL DIAGNOSIS

Haematemesis carries a mortality rate of 10% and is treated as a medical emergency. Consider the principle of Occam's razor here. There are many causes of haematemesis but the simplest explanation is likely to be the correct one (e.g. oesophageal varices in a chronic alcoholic; Mallory–Weiss tear after an alcohol binge; gastric erosions or a bleeding peptic ulcer in patients on long-term anti-inflammatories).

COMMON CAUSES OF HAEMATEMESIS

OESOPHAGITIS

- History of GORD (heartburn with acid brash)
- Fresh red blood with no red flag symptoms

GASTRIC/DUODENAL EROSION

- History of dyspepsia
- Associated with prolonged use of NSAIDs, steroids, SSRI or bisphosphonates

BLEEDING PEPTIC ULCER

- May present very unwell with peritonitis
- History of dyspepsia, nausea and smoking
- Associated with prolonged use of NSAIDs, steroids, SSRI or bisphosphonates

OESOPHAGEAL VARICES

- History of liver disease, possibly due to excessive alcohol consumption
- Bleeding can be extensive and catastrophic
- History of jaundice and/or known liver disease is likely to be given

UPPER GI MALIGNANCY

- Alarm symptoms – Anaemia, recent weight loss, poor appetite, recent onset of progressive symptoms, melaena and swallowing difficulty
- Early satiety is another feature of gastric carcinoma

MALLORY–WEISS TEAR

- Typically occurs after an uncontrollable bout of retching or coughing
- Fresh red blood with a history of excessive alcohol intake or eating disorders

RARER CAUSES

- Iatrogenic – Recent oesophageal/gastric surgery or endoscopy
- Arteriovenous malformations – Acute extensive haemorrhage; associated with hereditary haemorrhagic telangiectasia
- Boerhaave's syndrome – Oesophageal rupture due to excessive vomiting or retching; severe retrosternal and abdominal pain following vomiting; alcoholism present in 40% of patients
- Aorto-enteric fistula – Very rare condition, given some credence if the patient is known to have an abdominal aortic aneurysm or aortic graft in-situ

INVESTIGATIONS

- Check observations, perform abdominal and PR examination
- FBC, U&Es, LFTs, clotting, CRP, bone profile and group & save (if bleeding is minimal) or cross-match between two and four units (depending on severity)
- Erect chest x-ray – Free air under diaphragm indicates perforation
- Urgent upper GIT endoscopy
- CT abdomen/chest – For all patients with aortic grafts
- Angiography may be needed if source of bleeding not found at endoscopy

MANAGEMENT

Haematemesis should be treated as a medical emergency. Therefore, initial management should be completed in an ABCDE approach.

- Ensure airway is patent and secured. Use suction to remove any vomiting that could compromise airway.
- Assess respiratory rate and oxygen saturations. Give high-flow 15L oxygen via a non-rebreathe mask. Auscultate and percuss the chest.
- Assess character, rate and volume of pulse. Establish IV access and give IV fluids ± blood products to maintain circulation. Monitor blood pressure.
- Assess responsiveness with AVPU. Check pupils and blood glucose.
- Expose the patient. Check from head to toe for obvious signs of haemorrhage.

Always contact a senior doctor for support and ensure patients are kept nil by mouth for emergency endoscopy/surgery. Some hospitals use the *Rockall* score or the *Blatchford* score to stratify those with greatest need of urgent endoscopy.

Once the patient is stable, the following management can be used:

- Advice on alcohol intake and referral to alcohol specialist team for patients suffering from alcoholism
- Medication review to identify medications that could cause gastritis/ulcers such as NSAIDs, steroids, SSRIs and bisphosphonates
- Proton pump inhibitor cover for any patients on long-term NSAIDs/steroids
- 2-week referral for patients with suspected malignancy
- Treat positive *H. pylori* patients with triple therapy regime (usually two antibiotics and a proton pump inhibitor) as per local protocol

FURTHER READING

NICE guidance on upper GI bleeding, https://www.nice.org.uk/guidance/cg141/

CHANGE IN BOWEL HABIT (CONSTIPATION/DIARRHOEA IN ADULTS)

INITIATING THE SESSION

- Greet the patient, ask an open question and screen for other problems

MEDICAL PERSPECTIVE

SEQUENCE OF EVENTS

- **Open question** – Can you tell me more about what has been going on?
- **Timeline** – When did this start? How has it progressed?
- **Timing** – Has this happened before? *If so,* what happened then?

SYMPTOM ANALYSIS

- **Clarify** – When you say constipation/diarrhoea, what do you mean exactly? Do you mean you are going more/less often or the consistency has changed?
- **Frequency** – How many times a day do you open your bowels? How often is normal for you? What are your stools normally like? Do you ever suffer from the opposite? (i.e. constipation/diarrhoea)
- **Character/colour** – What are the stools like? Are they watery, semi-solid or solid? Is there any blood or mucus in the stools or on the tissue paper? What colour are they?
- **Melaena** – Do you get any dark foul-smelling stools?
- **Exacerbating/relieving factors** – Does anything trigger the constipation/diarrhoea? Does anything make it better?
- **Tenesmus** – Do you feel like you always need to go to the toilet, even after you've just been? Is this despite not passing very much stool?

SYSTEMS REVIEW

- **Abdominal pain** – Are you suffering from any abdominal pain?
- **Distension** – Do you tend to suffer from bloating and flatulence?
- **Upper GIT** – Any vomiting (*if so, ask about haematemesis*)? Any difficulties swallowing? Reflux or indigestion?
- **Constitutional** – Have you felt feverish? Have you lost any weight? How is your appetite? How have your energy levels been?
- **NS** – Have you had any back pain? Have you had any weakness in your legs?
- **Foreign travel** – Have you been abroad anywhere recently?

> **RED FLAGS**
> Anaemia (unexplained)
> Weight loss
> Age >60 years
> Rectal bleeding

PATIENT'S PERSPECTIVE

- **Feelings and effect on life** – How have your symptoms affected you?
- **Ideas** – Do you have any ideas yourself about what could be going on?
- **Concerns** – Is there anything you are particularly concerned could be causing your constipation/diarrhoea? Is there anything in general that concerns you?
- **Expectations** – Was there anything in particular you were hoping for today?

BACKGROUND INFORMATION

PMH

- Do you suffer from any medical conditions?
- *Ask specifically about anaemia, IBD and previous malignancy*

DH

- Do you take any regular medications? Any over-the-counter medications?
- *Ask specifically about laxatives/anti-diarrhoeals such as codeine*

FH

- Do any conditions run in the family?
- *Ask specifically about IBD and malignancy (colorectal and ovarian carcinoma – and determine which relatives they were and what age they were when they were diagnosed)*

SH

- Do you smoke? How many cigarettes do you smoke a day? For how long?
- Do you drink alcohol? How much do you drink in a week?
- Are you working presently? *If so,* what is your job? What does that involve?
- Can you tell me about your home situation (*occupants and any difficulties*)?
- Has your problem affected your job or home life in any way?

CLOSING THE SESSION

- summary ± examination/explanation and planning/contract

IMPORTANT POINTS

- Constipation and diarrhoea can mean different things to different people – make sure that you clarify early exactly what the patient means
- Quantify how many times they are going to the toilet and what affect it is having on their life
- Never forget to ask about red flag symptoms (e.g. cachexia, PR bleeding, anaemia and upper GIT symptoms)
- In lesions affecting the caecum/ascending colon there may be no change in bowel habit as faecal matter in this part of the colon is liquid/semi-solid (hence unexplained anaemia must be investigated), whereas lesions in the sigmoid colon/rectum will often cause a change in bowel habit due to obstruction
- Family history is very important here – do not forget!
- Symptoms of bloating and flatulence are often reported by patients, but they are of little clinical significance
- Interestingly, smoking exacerbates Crohn's disease, where as it appears to lower the risk of developing ulcerative colitis

DIFFERENTIAL DIAGNOSIS

FACTORS LIKELY TO CAUSE CONSTIPATION (MOST COMMON)

- Diet – Lack of fibre in diet; regular consumption of processed/ready-made meals; and reduced water intake
- Lack of exercise and immobility
- Medication – Opioids; iron supplements; amitriptyline; and many more
- Anorectal disease e.g. anal fissures that makes defecation a painful experience

COLORECTAL CANCER (MOST SERIOUS)

- Age over 55 years (unless familial predisposition mentioned)
- Red flag symptoms include cachexia, rectal bleeding, abdominal mass found and change in bowel habit lasting 6 weeks or more
- Always consider in men of any age or non-menstruating women with unexplained iron-deficiency anaemia
- Previous history of malignancy, IBD and coeliac disease

IBD

- Chronic diarrhoea with blood and mucus, and lower abdominal pain
- Fever, mouth ulcers, anorectal disease and extra-intestinal features may be present
- Consider in younger patients with above symptoms

IRRITABLE BOWEL SYNDROME

- Commoner in women (often young) and may be related to stress or anxiety
- Associated with bloating, constipation/diarrhoea and crampy abdominal pain
- No blood in the stools or other red flags present

GASTROENTERITIS

- Recent history of eating uncooked/poorly prepared food and/or foreign travel
- Diarrhoea (may be watery, bloody or simply loose) and vomiting
- Household members may also be unwell with similar symptoms

DIVERTICULAR DISEASE

- Middle-age/elderly patients with bloody diarrhoea and pain in left iliac fossa
- Can lead to diverticulitis, with fever, nausea and vomiting
- Risk factors include obesity and low dietary fibre

MALABSORPTION

- E.g. due to coeliac disease, chronic pancreatitis, thyroid disease or diabetes
- Steatorrhoea (pale offensive stools that are difficult to flush), weight loss and general malaise may accompany diarrhoea

OTHERS

- Overflow diarrhoea after constipation with faecal impaction
- Diabetic autonomic neuropathy
- Metabolic disturbance e.g. thyroid hormone and calcium abnormalities

INVESTIGATIONS

- Full abdominal examination and PR examination
- FBC – check for anaemia
- Other bloods: LFTs, U&Es, TFTs, CRP, ESR
- Stool culture
- Faecal occult blood test
- Abdominal x-ray
- Flexible sigmoidoscopy/colonoscopy and upper GIT endoscopy
- Abdominal CT scan

MANAGEMENT

- 2-week referral for patients with red flag symptoms
- Correct any electrolyte abnormalities and rehydrate the patient if necessary
- Advice on diet, hydration and lifestyle and medication review for constipation
- IBS – Dietary/lifestyle advice; antispasmodics; laxatives/anti-diarrhoeals; and psychological therapy
- IBD – Stop smoking (Crohn's); sulfasalazine (ulcerative colitis); infliximab in severe disease; surgery; steroids for flare-ups
- Gastroenteritis – Rehydration; antibiotics only if indicated by results of stool culture
- Diverticular disease – High-fibre diet and bulk-producing laxatives if no better
- Malabsorption – Treat underlying cause and give nutritional supplements

FURTHER READING

NICE CKS on:

    Diarrhoea in adults, http://cks.nice.org.uk/diarrhoea-adults-assessment

    Recognition of lower GIT cancers, http://cks.nice.org.uk/gastrointestinal-tract-lower-cancers-recognition-and-referral

JAUNDICE

INITIATING THE SESSION

- Greet the patient, ask an open question and screen for other problems

MEDICAL PERSPECTIVE

SEQUENCE OF EVENTS AND SYMPTOM ANALYSIS

- **Open question** – Can you tell me more about what has been going on?
- **Timeline** – When did this start? How has it progressed?
- **Timing** – Has this happened before? *If so,* what happened then?
- **Pruritus** – Have you noticed your skin become itchier?
- **Urine** – Has your urine become dark?
- **Steatorrhoea** – Have you developed pale greasy stools?

SYSTEMS REVIEW

- **Abdominal pain** – Do you have any pain in your abdomen?
- **Encephalopathy** – Have you become more confused?
- **Ascites** – Has your abdomen become more bloated or distended?
- **Constitutional** – Have you had any weight loss or loss of appetite? Any fever? Have you felt more tired than you would consider to be normal?
- **Rash** – Have you noticed any rash? Any bruising?
- **Foreign travel** – Have you been abroad in the past 6 months? *If so,* where?

> **RED FLAGS**
>
> *Confusion*
> *Haematemesis*
> *Fever*
> *Bruising/purpura*
> *Painless jaundice*
> *Weight loss*

ALCOHOL SCREENING HISTORY (INCLUDING CAGE QUESTIONNAIRE)

- How much alcohol do you drink in a week? Is this a typical week for you? Do you ever binge on alcohol? *If so,* how often do you tend to binge?
- **Cut down** – Have you ever felt you should cut down on your drinking?
- **Annoyed** – Have other people ever annoyed you by commenting on your drinking?
- **Guilt** – Have you ever felt guilty about the amount you drink?
- **Eye-opener** – Have you ever had a drink in the morning to settle yourself?

If answered yes to any of the CAGE questions, take a full alcohol history, see pp. 223

PATIENT'S PERSPECTIVE

- **Feelings and effect on life** – How do you feel about what has been going on? How have your symptoms affected your day-to-day life?
- **Ideas** – Do you have any ideas yourself about what could be going on?
- **Concerns** – Is there anything you are particularly concerned could be causing your symptoms? Is there anything in general that concerns you?
- **Expectations** – Was there anything in particular you were hoping for today?

BACKGROUND INFORMATION

PMH

- Do you suffer from any medical conditions? Do you have any problems with your liver?
- *Ask about liver disorders, previous cancer, surgery and autoimmune disorders*

DH

- Do you take any regular medications? Have any of them been changed recently?
- Do you have any allergies?

FH

- Do any conditions run in your family?
- Any family history of jaundice?

SH

- Do you smoke? How many cigarettes do you smoke a day? For how long?
- Have you ever used recreational drugs or self-injected?
- Are you working presently? *If so,* what is your job? What does that involve?
- Can you tell me about your home situation (*occupants and any difficulties*)?
- Has your problem affected your job or home life in any way?

CLOSING THE SESSION

- summary ± examination/explanation and planning/contract

IMPORTANT POINTS

- Jaundice (or icterus) is a term used to describe the yellow pigmentation of a patient's skin and sclerae caused by excess bilirubin in the blood. Jaundice normally becomes visible at bilirubin levels >35μmol/l
- It is very important to take a good alcohol history, as alcohol is one of the commonest pathological causes of jaundice
- Consider whether the patient has simply been unwell recently with a viral illness – Gilbert's syndrome is the commonest cause of jaundice and tends to be more pronounced during periods of illness
- An OSCE station may have either a simulated patient or perhaps a patient with long-standing jaundice from whom a focussed history is required

DIFFERENTIAL DIAGNOSIS

Jaundice is usually classified as pre-hepatic, hepatic or post-hepatic and a good history should establish which of these is most likely to be the underlying cause. Remember, jaundice may occasionally reflect a combination of both hepatic and post-hepatic causes. The key to the OSCE history is to identify whether the jaundice is pre-, intra- or post-hepatic and then to isolate the most likely aetiology. The differential diagnosis for jaundice is vast.

PRE-HEPATIC JAUNDICE

Unconjugated bilirubin is elevated in pre-hepatic jaundice. The patient does not develop pale stools or dark urine.

GILBERT'S SYNDROME (MOST COMMON)

- Congenital hyperbilirubinaemia present in 5% of population
- Often present with jaundice at time of any viral illness
- Crigler–Najjar syndrome is another more severe congenital hyperbilirubinaemia

MALARIA

- Transmitted by mosquitos after travel to an endemic area
- Fever, myalgia, headache, malaise at least 6 days after transmission

HAEMOLYSIS

- Abnormal breakdown of red blood cells
- Can be due to an inherited condition (e.g. G6PD deficiency) autoimmune haemolytic anaemia, hypersplenism and various other less common causes

HEPATOCELLULAR JAUNDICE

Both unconjugated and conjugated bilirubin can be elevated in pre-hepatic jaundice. Pale urine and dark stools may be present in hepatocellular jaundice.

HEPATITIS

- Alcoholic hepatitis
- Viral hepatitis A (contaminated food), B and C (sexual contact; IVDU), infectious mononucleosis ("kissing disease")
- Drug-induced hepatitis e.g. from paracetamol overdose
- Autoimmune hepatitis

HEPATOCELLULAR CARCINOMA

- Most commonly secondary to chronic hepatitis B or C infection
- Can be secondary to alcoholic hepatitis, primary biliary cirrhosis and hereditary haemochromatosis

METASTATIC DISEASE FROM OTHER PRIMARY SITE (MOST SERIOUS)

- Colorectal, lung, breast, pancreatic, stomach, melanoma and neuroendocrine cancers are the most common types that spread to the liver

OTHER CAUSES

- Wilson's disease
- Hereditary haemochromatosis
- Hepatic congestion from cardiac failure

POST-HEPATIC JAUNDICE

Conjugated bilirubin is elevated in post-hepatic jaundice. Pale stools and dark urine are features due to the absence of bile salts being released into the digestive system to absorb fats and the presence of conjugated bilirubin in the urine, respectively.

PANCREATIC CARCINOMA (MOST SERIOUS)

- Painless jaundice from obstruction of biliary tree by the head of the pancreas
- Poor prognosis

GALLSTONES

- Common in females; those aged near 40 years; and obese
- Painful
- Only cause jaundice if they obstruct the common bile duct

OTHER CAUSES

- Porta hepatis lymph nodes
- Primary biliary cirrhosis
- Primary sclerosing cholangitis

INVESTIGATIONS

- Bloods including FBC, LFTs, U+Es, full liver screen (including viral serology and autoimmune screen), paracetamol level and blood film for malaria
- Liver USS ± CT abdomen
- MRCP for gallstones
- Biopsy

MANAGEMENT

- No treatment required for Gilbert's syndrome
- Antibiotics for malaria
- Antiviral therapy for viral hepatitis
- Cessation of alcohol consumption in alcoholic liver disease
- Acetylcysteine for paracetamol overdose
- Regular phlebotomy for haemochromatosis
- Caeruloplasmin for Wilson's disease

- Cholecystectomy and ERCP for gallstones causing bile duct obstruction
- Surgery, chemotherapy and radiotherapy for hepatic and pancreatic cancer depending on extent and metastatic involvement

FURTHER READING

NICE CKS on jaundice, http://cks.nice.org.uk/jaundice-in-adults

Neurology

4

COLLAPSE AND SEIZURES

INITIATING THE SESSION

- Greet the patient, ask an open question and screen for other problems

MEDICAL PERSPECTIVE

SEQUENCE OF EVENTS AND SYMPTOM ANALYSIS

Before

- **Open question** – Can you talk me through what happened exactly? What were you doing at the time? What do you think caused you to collapse?
- **Preceding symptoms** – How did you feel immediately before the episode? Did you have any warning that something was about to happen? Any headache? Any strange vision or sensations? Any chest pain? Any palpitations? Any difficulty breathing?
- **Witness** – Did anyone witness the episode? How did they describe the episode?

During

- **Fall** – How did you fall exactly? Did you hit your head?
- **LOC** – Did you lose consciousness? *If so*, for how long?
- **Seizure** – Did you have a fit? *If so*, can you describe it? Did your whole body shake or only part of it?
- **Continence** – Did you pass any urine or soil yourself?
- **Tongue** – Did you bite your tongue? *If yes*, was it the front or the side?
- **Complexion** – Did anyone notice your face change colour before you collapsed?

After

- **Post-ictal state** – How did you feel immediately after the fall/when you regained consciousness? Were you confused? Drowsy? Aching muscles?
- **Todd's paralysis** – Did you have any weakness afterwards?

- **Previous episodes** – Has something like this ever happened before? *If yes,* can you describe exactly what happened those times?

SYSTEMS REVIEW

- **NS** – Do you have any weakness in your muscles now? Any strange sensations or numbness? How is your vision? How is your balance?
- **RS/CVS** – Have you had any chest pain? Any palpitations? A cough? Any shortness of breath?
- **GIT** – Have you had any abdominal pain recently? Has your bowel habit changed? Any bleeding from the back passage?
- **GUT** – Have you noticed any blood in the urine?
- **Constitutional** – Have you noticed any significant weight loss recently? Any night sweats? Any lumps anywhere? Any fever?

PATIENT'S PERSPECTIVE

- **Effect on life** – How have these blackouts affected your daily life? Are you driving?
- **Feelings** – How do you feel about what happened?
- **Ideas** – What do you think caused the blackout?
- **Concerns** – Are you concerned anything else could be going on? Is there anything in general that is concerning you?
- **Expectations** – When you made the appointment, other than getting my opinion, was there anything in particular you were hoping for?

BACKGROUND INFORMATION

PMH

- Do you suffer from any medical conditions?
- *Ask specifically about epilepsy and arrhythmias*

DH

- Are you taking any medications? Any allergies?

FH

- Do any conditions run in your family?
- Has anyone in your family died young unexpectedly from a heart condition?

SH

- How much alcohol do you drink? Had you been drinking at the time of the blackout?
- Do you smoke?
- Do you take any recreational drugs?
- Are you working presently? *If so,* what is your job? What does that involve?
- Can you tell me about your home situation (*occupants and any difficulties*)?
- Has your problem affected your job or home life in any way?

CLOSING THE SESSION

- summary ± examination/explanation and planning/contract

> **IMPORTANT POINTS**
>
> - It is important to verify if anyone else witnessed the episode and make it clear that you would like to get their story of events
> - A detailed description of the episode is crucial – subtle differences will help distinguish an epileptic seizure from syncopal episodes and arrhythmias
> - Always consider the damage the fall has done as well – did they hit their head and is there any indication of trauma elsewhere?
> - In elderly patients with cognitive impairment and where it is not clear whether or not it was truly a collapse, it can be important to focus more on the social side of the history (*see falls history, pp. 6*)

DIFFERENTIAL DIAGNOSIS

VASOVAGAL SYNCOPE/COMMON FAINT (MOST COMMON)

- "3 Ps" – Posture (prolonged standing), provoking factors and prodromal symptoms
- Evoked by strong emotion (e.g. fear) and pain
- Nausea, pallor, feeling hot and sweaty often precede episode by a few seconds
- Brief loss of consciousness, lasting seconds usually
- Limb jerking is uncommon and there should be no post-ictal state

CARDIOGENIC SYNCOPE (MOST SERIOUS)

- Aortic stenosis/acute coronary syndrome – Central chest pain and dyspnoea
- Stokes–Adams attack – Collapse without warning, appearing pale with a slow or absent pulse and rapid recovery with facial flushing; LOC 10–30 seconds; may be due to heart block from a myocardial infarction

SEIZURE

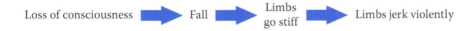

Loss of consciousness → Fall → Limbs go stiff → Limbs jerk violently

- Aura may precede episode (visual; olfactory; sensory; déjà-vu)
- Biting side of tongue and urinary/faecal incontinence
- A post-ictal state of drowsiness, myalgia, headache and amnesia is common
- Can last up to 2–3 minutes

SITUATIONAL SYNCOPE

- Micturition (particularly men at night) or a coughing attack may precipitate syncope

CAROTID SINUS SYNCOPE

- Turning of the head or shaving can lead to brief loss of consciousness

POSTURAL HYPOTENSION

- Often after the patient moves from a lying/sitting position to standing
- Very brief episode (lasting a few seconds) following a "head rush" or unsteadiness
- Anti-cholinergic medications e.g. tricyclic antidepressants or anti-hypertensive medications may contribute

INVESTIGATIONS

- Full cardiovascular and neurological examination
- Bloods – FBC, full electrolyte screen, cardiac enzymes if suspecting ACS
- ECG – acute coronary syndrome and arrhythmias
- 24- or 72-hour ECG monitoring – Transient arrhythmia e.g. Stokes–Adam's attack
- Lying and standing blood pressure – Drop of >20/10 mm Hg = postural hypotension
- CT head for first seizure or if worrying features or neurological signs
- Echocardiogram – Aortic stenosis; hypertrophic obstructive cardiomyopathy in young

MANAGEMENT

- If the story is typical of vasovagal syncope with no red flags, then reassure the patient
- Where no clear cause is found on initial assessment you should consider admitting the patient for the investigations above
- Advise the patient they should not be driving until seen by a specialist and to inform the DVLA if they have had a blackout not due to an uncomplicated faint
- Advise the patient to take precautions (e.g. not bathing alone), in case a similar episode happens again to put them at risk
- Advise the patient to record any future events on video if possible to aid diagnosis
- Refer to neurology for seizures for consideration of anti-epileptic therapy
- If recurrent seizures, educate and consider therapy
- If syncope provoked by exercise, advise the patient to avoid exercise until assessed by a cardiologist
- Treat myocardial infarction, aortic stenosis and any arrhythmias appropriately
- In postural hypotension, review medications and avoid precipitating factors (e.g. tell patients to get up slowly and carefully)

REFERENCE

1. NICE head injury guidance, https://www.nice.org.uk/guidance/cg176

FURTHER READING

NICE guidance on loss of consciousness, https://www.nice.org.uk/guidance/cg109

HEADACHE

INITIATING THE SESSION

- Greet the patient, ask an open question and screen for other problems

MEDICAL PERSPECTIVE

SEQUENCE OF EVENTS

- **Open question** – Can you tell me more about these headaches?
- **Timeline** – How did the headache start? How have your symptoms progressed since?

SYMPTOM ANALYSIS (SOCRATES)

- **Site** – Where exactly do you feel the pain? Can you point to the area?
- **Onset** – Did it come on suddenly? Do you have any warnings prior to the headache?
- **Character** – Was it one episode or multiple? Describe the pain.
- **Radiation** – Does the pain move anywhere else?
- **Associated symptoms** – *See systems review*
- **Timing** – When can you remember this starting? Was it continuous or intermittent? How long do they last? When was the last time you had a headache?
- **Exacerbating or relieving factors** – Does it get worse on coughing? Is it worse at night or in the early morning? Any particular activities or movements? Does anything relieve the pain?
- **Severity** – How bad was the pain on a scale of 1–10 initially, with 10 being the worst pain you can imagine? How about now? Is it painful to touch or press over anywhere?

SYSTEMS REVIEW

- **Trauma** – Have you fallen and hit your head recently?
- **Constitutional** – Have you felt unwell or feverish? Have you lost any weight? Any nausea or vomiting?
- **Meningism** – Are you sensitive to light? Do you have any neck stiffness? Have you noticed a rash anywhere?
- **NS** – Have you had any arm or leg weakness? Any visual disturbances? Any other sensory disturbance?
- **Aura** – Did you have any strange symptoms before the headache came on, such as visual disturbance, numbness or otherwise?
- **Seizures/blackouts** – Have you ever had seizures or blacked out?
- **Sentinel headache** – *If acute,* have you had a less severe headache recently?
- **MS** – Is it painful to comb your hair or to chew? Do you have any visual changes? Do you have any pain or aches in your shoulders?

> **RED FLAGS**
>
> Meningism
> Non-blanching rash
> Systemically unwell
> Weight loss
> Neurological symptoms
> Seizures
> Age >65 years and
>   unilateral

PATIENT'S PERSPECTIVE

- **Effect on life** – How have these headaches affected your daily life?
- **Feelings** – How do you feel about the headaches? Have they affected your mood?

- **Ideas** – What do you think is causing the headaches?
- **Concerns** – Some people who get headaches worry it could be cancer. Is that something that concerns you? Is there anything else that is concerning you?
- **Expectations** – When you made the appointment, other than getting my opinion, was there anything in particular you were hoping for?

BACKGROUND INFORMATION

PMH

- Do you suffer from any other medical conditions?
- Have you ever had headache like this before? *If so,* what was the cause?

DH

- Are you taking any medications? Do you have any allergies?

FH

- Do any conditions run in your family?

SH

- How much alcohol do you drink?
- Do you smoke? How many do/did you smoke? For how many years?
- Are you working presently? *If so,* what is your job? What does that involve?
- Can you tell me about your home situation (*occupants and any difficulties*)?
- Has your problem affected your job or home life in any way?

CLOSING THE SESSION

- summary ± examination/explanation and planning/contract

IMPORTANT POINTS

- After asking open questions, it is best to characterise headache first into whether it is unilateral or bilateral, the kind of pain involved and associated symptoms to gain a quick idea of which line of questioning to take
- It is important to exclude potentially life-threatening causes by asking about red flag symptoms
- Never forget to consider emergencies such as subarachnoid or extradural haemorrhage, meningitis, temporal arteritis, angle closure glaucoma, raised intracranial pressure and subdural haemorrhage. These can be more easily memorised by starting in the brain parenchyma (tumour), then the vessels (haemorrhage and clots), then the meninges (meningitis), then extracranial arteries (temporal arteritis) and finally the eye (glaucoma)

DIFFERENTIAL DIAGNOSIS

One of the first things to consider is whether the headache is recurring or happening for the first time. Headaches occurring for the first time obviously could still be migraine, cluster headaches or tension headaches, but it is important to try to rule out sinister causes.

FIRST HEADACHE

MENINGITIS

- Classical presentation – Headache, fever, neck stiffness and photophobia
- Non-blanching purpuric rash indicates meningococcal septicaemia
- Later presentation includes seizures, decreased conscious level and even coma

EXTRADURAL HAEMORRHAGE

- Typically, due to trauma to the temple, damaging the middle meningeal artery
- There may be a lucid interval, with increasingly severe headache, associated raised ICP symptoms and gradually decreasing consciousness until complete loss

SUBDURAL HAEMORRHAGE

- Common in the elderly after falling/banging their head in previous weeks/months
- Worsening pain, decreasing consciousness, increased sleepiness and ataxia
- ICP gradually increases until it causes symptoms (*see below*)

SUBARACHNOID HAEMORRHAGE

- Sudden, severe "thunderclap" headache, sometimes with a sentinel headache of less severity within the weeks prior to the current headache
- Meningism e.g. neck stiffness and photophobia
- Linked to polycystic kidney disease and Ehlers–Danlos syndrome

RAISED INTRACRANIAL PRESSURE

- Often described as "worst headache ever"
- Morning headache, worse on coughing, lying down or any valsalva manoeuvre
- May have visual disturbances, seizures and other neurological symptoms

TEMPORAL ARTERITIS

- Severe headache located in the temple area
- Jaw claudication, scalp tenderness; often polymyalgia rheumatic symptoms
- Sudden blindness in one eye if not treated promptly

ACUTE SINUSITIS

- Constant dull ache worse on bending forward, associated with coryzal symptoms
- Often followed by purulent rhinorrhoea/productive cough as sinuses clear

OTHERS

- Angle closure glaucoma – Acute painful red eye, visual halos, reduced vision
- Medication – Mixed analgesics may cause a headache themselves
- Trigeminal neuralgia – Short, intense "electric shock" pain in trigeminal nerve distribution triggered by touching affected area (e.g. shaving or brushing hair)

RECURRENT HEADACHE

MIGRAINE

- Severe, pulsating, recurring, unilateral headache that lasts around an hour
- Often has visual or sensory "aura," occurring shortly before onset
- Photophobia/phonophobia when headache starts, patient seeks dark quiet room
- Triggers – Changes in diet, oral contraceptives, exercise, caffeine and alcohol

CLUSTER HEADACHE

- Excruciating, recurring, unilateral headache normally localised around one eye
- Lasts for only a few hours, often twice in 24 hours and most common at night
- Headaches occur in clusters for weeks, then headache-free for months
- Associated with profuse eye watering and nasal secretions on the affected side

TENSION HEADACHE

- Bilateral and associated with stress and visual strain (reading, watching TV)
- Typically described as a tight band across the head that lasts minutes to hours
- No other signs or symptoms

INVESTIGATIONS

- Neurological examination and examination for tender areas over skull
- Ophthalmoscopy (for evidence of papilloedema)
- Bloods – FBC, U&Es, CRP and ESR
- Temporal artery biopsy if temporal arteritis suspected
- CT/MRI scan
- Lumbar puncture if not contraindicated

MANAGEMENT

- General – Analgesia and hydration; ABCDE approach if acutely unwell
- Migraine – Avoid precipitants; triptan (e.g. sumatriptan) when headache starts
- Cluster headache – 100% oxygen and sumatriptan for acute attacks; verapamil or prednisolone for prophylaxis
- Meningitis – IV antibiotics (e.g. cefotaxime)
- Intracranial haemorrhage – Neurosurgery (e.g. craniotomy plus evacuation)

- Raised ICP – Elevate head of bed to 30 degrees; sedation, cerebrospinal fluid drainage, mannitol, neuromuscular blockade and hyperventilation lower ICP
- Temporal arteritis – High-dose oral prednisolone, arrange temporal artery biopsy and urgent rheumatology referral

FURTHER READING

NICE guidance on headache assessment, http://cks.nice.org.uk/headache-assessment

WEAKNESS

INITIATING THE SESSION

- Greet the patient, ask an open question and screen for other problems

MEDICAL PERSPECTIVE

SEQUENCE OF EVENTS

- **Open question** – Can you tell me exactly what you have noticed?
- **Timeline** – How did it start? How have your symptoms progressed since then?

SYMPTOM ANALYSIS (SOCRATES)

- **Site** – Where is the weakness? Legs? Arms? Facial muscles? One side or both?
- **Onset** – When did you first notice it? Did it come on suddenly or gradually? *If suddenly, what were you doing at the time?*
- **Character** – Is the weakness always there or does it vary?
- **Radiation** – Do you have weakness anywhere else?
- **Associated features** – *See systems review*
- **Timing** – Has it ever happened before?
- **Exacerbating/relieving factors** – Does anything make it better or worse? Do your muscles tire easily?
- **Severity** – How bad is the weakness? Do you have any movement? Are you able to walk/ use your arms?

SYSTEMS REVIEW

- **Sensory** – Do you have any numbness or tingling anywhere? Have you noticed any changes in your vision? Hearing? Taste? Smell?
- **Muscle wasting** – Have you noticed a reduction in muscle bulk in the areas affected?
- **Balance** – Any problems with your balance?
- **Speech** – Have you had any trouble with your speech previously?
- **Headaches** – Have you had any bad headaches recently? *If so, SOCRATES*
- **Seizures and blackouts** – Have you had any seizures or blackouts?
- **Pain** – Have you had any back pain or pain elsewhere? *If so, SOCRATES*
- **Incontinence** – Have you had any trouble controlling your waterworks or bowels?
- **Constitutional** – Have you felt ill or feverish recently? Have you noticed any weight loss? How has your appetite been? Have you been feeling tired?

PATIENT'S PERSPECTIVE

- **Feelings and effect on life** – How has all of this affected your daily life?
- **Ideas** – What do you think is causing the weakness?
- **Concerns** – Is there anything in particular you are worried could be causing it? Is there anything in general that is concerning you about the weakness?
- **Expectations** – When you made the appointment, other than getting my opinion, was there anything in particular you were hoping for?

BACKGROUND INFORMATION

PMH

- Do you suffer from any medical conditions?

DH

- Are you taking any medications? Do you have any allergies?

FH

- Do any conditions run in your family?
- *Ask specifically about muscular dystrophy*

SH

- Are you working presently? *If so,* what is your job? What does that involve?
- Can you tell me about your home situation (*occupants and any difficulties*)?
- How has your problem affected your job and home life?
- Do you drink alcohol? How much do you drink in a week?
- Do you smoke? How many do/did you smoke? For how many years?

CLOSING THE SESSION

- summary ± examination/explanation and planning/contract

> **IMPORTANT POINTS**
>
> - It is important to clarify exactly which parts of the body are affected by the weakness – Upper/lower limbs; left/right; proximal/distal muscles as this will help aid diagnosis
> - During the history, you should be trying to localise where the problem lies – Does it lie in the muscles, neuromuscular junction, peripheral nerve, plexus, nerve root, spinal cord or the brain?
> - The nature of the weakness will provide many clues – Muscles that quickly fatigue and lose power may indicate myasthenia gravis, whereas an acute onset of muscle weakness affecting only one side is typical of a stroke

DIFFERENTIAL DIAGNOSIS

There are seven broad areas that can cause symptoms of weakness. If you split your history taking up with these in mind, it may help – Muscle, neuromuscular junction, peripheral nerve, plexus, nerve root, spinal cord and the brain.

MUSCLES

MUSCULAR DYSTROPHY (E.G. DUCHENNE'S AND BECKER'S MUSCULAR DYSTROPHY)

- Onset usually during childhood
- Painless gradual weakness predominantly affecting proximal limb muscles
- Difficultly standing up/walking

POLYMYOSITIS/DERMATOMYOSITIS

- Slow onset proximal muscle weakness and myalgia – Difficultly standing up/walking
- Fever, subcutaneous calcifications, Raynaud's phenomenon and interstitial lung disease may be present
- Dermatomyositis involves skin – Cracked dry skin on hands; heliotrope rash around eyes; macular rash ("shawl sign" over the shoulders); Gottron's papules over knuckles

MUSCLE WASTING FROM DISUSE

- Patients who are bedbound for a period of time
- Patients who have had a limb cast

NEUROMUSCULAR JUNCTION

MYASTHENIA GRAVIS

- Autoimmune condition in which patients' muscles become weak after use
- Often affects face, eye movement and eyelid muscles most
- Also causes a proximal myopathy with symptoms worse at end of the day
- Thymoma often present

LAMBERT–EATON MYASTHENIC SYNDROME

- Paraneoplastic syndrome that unlike myasthenia gravis spares the eyes
- Patients' weakness improves on repeated use of the muscle
- Autonomic dysfunction

PERIPHERAL NERVES (*See altered sensation pp. 74*)

- Peripheral neuropathy
- Mononeuropathy
- Mononeuritis multiplex

SPINAL CORD (*See altered sensation pp. 74*)

- Radiculopathy/plexopathy
- Cervical spondylosis
- Syringomyelia
- Spinal stenosis

CENTRAL (*See altered sensation pp. 74*)

- Multiple sclerosis
- Stroke
- Tumour/abscess

MOTOR NEURON DISEASE

- Gradual loss of upper and lower motor neurones
- Limb weakness (e.g. dropping objects and/or "heavy" legs), speech problems, dysphagia and dyspnoea; but no sensory or sphincter loss
- Often >40 y/o
- Difficulties with activities of daily living
- Rule out other causes of weakness first

INVESTIGATIONS

- Full neurological examination (lower limb, upper limb and cranial nerves)
- Bloods – FBC, U&Es, creatine kinase, autoimmune screen
- Chest x-ray
- Nerve conduction studies
- Tensillon test for myasthenia gravis
- CT/MRI brain/spinal cord/both (depending on clinical findings)

MANAGEMENT

- Encourage physical activity and offer physiotherapy
- Muscular dystrophy – Support, genetic counselling; orthoses and prednisolone may help prolong ambulatory phase
- Polymyositis – Immunosuppression with oral prednisolone
- Myasthenia gravis – Acetylcholinesterase inhibitors, immunosuppression with steroids and/or steroid-sparing agents; thymectomy
- Motor neuron disease – Palliative care through a multidisciplinary approach, including physiotherapy, speech and language therapy, occupational therapy and gastrostomy for dysphagia; riluzole may prolong life by around 3 months
- Others – *See altered sensation pp. 74*

FURTHER READING

NICE CKS on CNS cancer recognition, http://cks.nice.org.uk/brain-and-central-nervous-system-cancers-recognition-and-referral

ALTERED SENSATION

INITIATING THE SESSION

- Greet the patient, ask an open question and screen for other problems

MEDICAL PERSPECTIVE

SEQUENCE OF EVENTS

- **Open question** – Can you tell me exactly what you have noticed?
- **Timeline** – How did it start? How have your symptoms progressed since then?

SYMPTOM ANALYSIS (SOCRATES)

- **Site** – Where do you get this feeling? Does it affect both sides of the body?
- **Onset** – When did you first notice this? Did it come on suddenly or gradually?
- **Character** – Can you describe what it feels like exactly?
- **Radiation** – Do you have the same sensation anywhere else?
- **Associated factors** – *See systems review*
- **Timing** – Is it there all the time or does it come and go?
- **Exacerbating/relieving factors** – What, if anything, brings it on? Is it worse with stress? Heat? Exercise?
- **Severity** – How is it affecting you day-to-day?

SYSTEMS REVIEW

- **Sensory** – Have you had any changes in vision or eye pain? Any blurred vision in hot temperatures? Any change in your hearing? Taste? Smell?
- **Motor** – Have you noticed any muscle weakness anywhere?
- **Balance** – Any problems with your balance?
- **Speech** – Have you had any trouble with your speech previously?
- **Headaches** – Have you had any bad headaches recently? *If so, SOCRATES*
- **Seizures and blackouts** – Have you had any seizures or blackouts?
- **Pain** – Have you had any back pain or pain elsewhere? *If so, SOCRATES*
- **Incontinence** – Have you had any trouble controlling your waterworks or bowels?
- **Constitutional** – Have you felt feverish? Any weight loss? Have you been feeling more tired than you would consider normal?
- **Anxiety** – Do you panic or feel anxious each time before it happens?
- **Vascular** – Does it happen when your hands or feet are cold? Do your hands/feet turn white, then blue, then red? Is it painful when they are red?

PATIENT'S PERSPECTIVE

- **Feelings and effect on life** – How has this affected your daily life?
- **Ideas** – What do you think is causing your symptoms?
- **Concerns** – Is there anything in particular you are concerned could be causing it? Is there anything in general that is concerning you?
- **Expectations** – When you made the appointment, other than getting my opinion, was there anything in particular you were hoping for?

BACKGROUND INFORMATION

PMH

- Do you suffer from any medical conditions?

DH

- Are you taking any medications? Do you have any allergies?

FH

- Do any conditions run in your family?

SH

- Are you working presently? *If so,* what is your job? What does that involve?
- Can you tell me about your home situation (*occupants and any difficulties*)?
- Has your problem affected your job or home life in any way?
- Do you drink alcohol? How much do you drink in a week? Is this a typical week? (*Ask CAGE questions if considering alcohol as a cause of neuropathy*)
- Do you smoke? How many do/did you smoke? For how many years?

CLOSING THE SESSION

- summary ± examination/explanation and planning/contract

> **IMPORTANT POINTS**
> - The key to this history is to differentiate between a pathological cause of paraesthesia and a supra-tentorial cause. This can be challenging.
> - Beware of the patient who describes numbness "all over."
> - During the history, you should be trying to localise where the problem lies – Does it lie in the muscles, neuromuscular junction, peripheral nerve, plexus, nerve root, spinal cord or the brain?

DIFFERENTIAL DIAGNOSIS

CENTRAL

Multiple sclerosis

- Demyelinating disorder diagnosed by clinical, laboratory or radiological evidence of central nervous system lesions disseminated in time and space
- Common presentations – Optic neuritis, altered sensation, weakness and ataxia
- INSULAR – Intention tremor; Nystagmus; Slurred speech; Urogenital symptoms; Labile emotions; Ataxia; Retrobulbar neuritis

Stroke/transient ischaemic attack

- Sudden onset, affecting any part(s) of the central nervous system
- Other neurological symptoms likely e.g. motor, speech and eyesight problems

Tumour/abscess

- Slowly evolving symptoms such as seizures, focal neurological deficits, cognitive/personality changes and signs of raised ICP (*see headache history*)

SPINAL CORD

Radiculopathy/plexopathy

- Pressure on nerve root affecting sensory or motor modalities from that root
- Meralgia paraesthetica – A common benign complaint of thigh numbness due to irritation of the lateral cutaneous nerve of the thigh
- Shingles causes intense pain and blistering in a dermatomal distribution

Cervical spondylosis

- Altered sensation below level affected; neck stiffness possible
- Upper limbs – LMN signs
- Lower limbs – UMN signs

Spinal stenosis

- Pressure on spine from mass, trauma or spondylolisthesis
- Sensory level with altered sensation below affected level
- LMN signs at affected level, with UMN signs below affected level

Syringomyelia

- Specific area of sensory or motor loss related to location of syrinx
- Usually one sensory tract is lost at a time e.g. spinothalamic tract
- Symptoms may worsen due to events such as trauma, sneezing or coughing

PERIPHERAL NEUROPATHY

Mononeuropathy – e.g. Due to trauma, carpal tunnel syndrome or infection

- Affects a single dermatome and/or myotome; can be motor, sensory or both
- Can happen following trauma/nerve compression e.g. pressure on the medial epicondyle of the humerus may lead to ulnar nerve palsy
- Carpal tunnel syndrome – Pain and numbness in median nerve distribution; typically, at night, with patient waking and shaking their hand to relieve it

Mononeuritis multiplex – e.g. Due to diabetes, autoimmune infections or amyloidosis

- Inflammation of multiple single peripheral nerves, causing pain, numbness and weakness, associated with the above conditions

Polyneuropathy

- Causes (ABCDE) – Alcohol, vitamin B deficiency, chronic renal failure, diabetes and everything else (e.g. multiple sclerosis, cancer, amyloidosis)
- Can be mainly motor or sensory ("glove and stocking distribution") or mixed

NON-NEUROLOGICAL CAUSES

Anxiety attacks (± hyperventilation)

- History of anxiety with tingling sensations around mouth and in fingers
- Sympathetic response – Tachycardia, sweating, trembling and/or shaking

Raynaud's phenomenon

- Hands turn from white to blue to red (with severe pain), often when cold
- Primary Raynaud's is very common and benign; secondary causes include autoimmune conditions e.g. scleroderma and lupus – Distal necrosis/ulcers

INVESTIGATIONS

- Neurological examination
- Bloods – FBC, U&Es, vitamin levels, HbA1C (if diabetic), gamma-GT
- Nerve conduction studies
- CT/MRI brain/spinal cord/both (depending on clinical findings)

MANAGEMENT

- Multiple sclerosis – Symptomatic treatment (e.g. analgesia); steroids for flare-ups; azathioprine and interferon may be considered to reduce relapses
- Stroke – Early intervention imperative; aspirin initially; thrombolysis in ischaemic stroke; neurosurgery in haemorrhagic stroke
- Treat underlying cause of peripheral neuropathies e.g. carpal tunnel syndrome – local steroid injection or carpal tunnel release surgery if problematic

FURTHER READING

NICE CKS on:

    Neuropathic pain, http://cks.nice.org.uk/neuropathic-pain-drug-treatment
    Multiple sclerosis, http://cks.nice.org.uk/multiple-sclerosis
    Stroke, http://cks.nice.org.uk/stroke-and-tia

Musculoskeletal medicine

BACK PAIN

INITIATING THE SESSION

- Greet the patient, ask an open question and screen for other problems

MEDICAL PERSPECTIVE

SEQUENCE OF EVENTS

- **Open question** – Can you tell me more about your back pain?
- **Timeline** – How did the pain start? How has the pain progressed since then?

SYMPTOM ANALYSIS (SOCRATES)

- **Site** – Where exactly do you feel the pain? Can you point to the area?
- **Onset** – When did you first notice the pain? Did it come on suddenly or gradually?
- **Character** – What is the pain like?
- **Radiation** – Does the pain go anywhere else? Does it travel down your legs? *If so, how far?*
- **Associated features** – *See systems review*
- **Timing** – Is the pain always there or does it come and go? Is it worse at any particular time of the day?
- **Exacerbating/relieving factors** – Does anything make the pain better or worse? Is it made better or worse by movement? Is it made better or worse by rest? Does the pain ever wake you up at night? Have you tried taking any painkillers for it?
- **Severity** – If you had to score the pain between 1 and 10 with 10 being the worst pain you can imagine, how would you score your pain?

SYSTEMS REVIEW

- **Trauma** – Was there any history of trauma?
- **NS** – Have your legs been feeling weaker than usual? Have you had any strange sensations down your legs or buttocks? Have you had any problems controlling your waterworks or bowels?

RED FLAGS

New onset incontinence
Saddle anaesthesia
Muscle weakness in legs
History of cancer
Weight loss
Non-mechanical
Night-time pain
Violent trauma
Age <20 or >50 years
Thoracic back pain
Intravenous drug use

- **MS** – Is your back stiff in the morning? *If so*, how long does that last for? Do you have pains in any other joints?
- **Constitutional** – Have you noticed any weight loss over the past few months? How is your appetite? Have you been feeling feverish or ill recently? How has your mood been?

PATIENT'S PERSPECTIVE

- **Feelings and effect on life** – How has your back pain affected your daily life?
- **Ideas** – What do you think is causing the back pain?
- **Concerns** – Is there anything in particular you are concerned could be causing it? Is there anything in general that is concerning you about the back pain?
- **Expectations** – When you make the appointment, other than getting my opinion, was there anything in particular you were hoping for?

BACKGROUND INFORMATION

PMH

- Do you have any medical conditions? Have you suffered from back pain before?
- *Ask specifically about osteoporosis, arthritis and previous cancer*

DH

- Are you currently taking any medications? Do you have any allergies?

FH

- Do any conditions run in the family?
- Has anyone in your family had trouble with back pain?
- *Ask specifically about ankylosing spondylitis and osteoporosis*

SH

- Are you working presently? *If so*, what is your job? What does that involve?
- Can you tell me about your home situation (*occupants and any difficulties*)?
- Has your problem affected your job or home life in any way?
- Do you smoke? How many do you smoke a day? How many years for?
- Do you drink alcohol? How much do you drink in a week?
- Do you use any recreational drugs? *Look for intravenous drugs use*

CLOSING THE SESSION

- summary ± examination/explanation and planning/contract

IMPORTANT POINTS

- Always enquire about red flag symptoms to rule out sinister causes
- Cord compression and cauda equina are medical emergencies and must be sought after in the history

- Ruptured and dissected aortic aneurysms commonly present with severe back/loin pain in patients (site of pain dependent on site of rupture or dissection)
- The patient's perspective and social history are very important as chronic back pain is one of the commonest causes of long-term disability and sickness
- Chronic back pain is defined as that lasting longer than 6 weeks

YELLOW FLAG SYMPTOMS (PROGNOSTIC OF LONG-TERM DISABILITY):
- Negative attitude that their back pain is severely disabling
- Belief that activity is harmful to recovery
- Belief that passive treatment will be beneficial
- Depression and social withdrawal
- Financial difficulties

DIFFERENTIAL DIAGNOSIS

COMMON

Mechanical/non-specific lower back pain (most common)

- Clinical diagnosis in the absence of red flags where the pain varies with posture and is worse on movement
- There will frequently be a history of previous similar episodes over a number of years
- There may be a history of mild trauma/heavy lifting or it could be spontaneous

Radiculopathy (sciatica)

- Unilateral leg pain radiating below the knee to the foot or toes
- Leg pain may be worse than the back pain

SERIOUS

Cauda equina syndrome (most serious)

- Urinary and faecal incontinence
- Sensory numbness of buttocks and backs of thighs and weakness of legs
- The most common causes are malignancy and infection

Malignancy

- Systemically unwell (e.g. weight loss) and symptoms from primary malignancy
- Usually of gradual onset, with constant pain not relieved by rest
- History of malignancy with tendency to metastasise to bone, such as multiple myeloma, prostatic or breast carcinoma

Osteoporotic crush fracture

- Risk factors for osteoporosis include increasing age, female, corticosteroid therapy, premature menopause (<40 years), smoking and malabsorption
- Sudden localised back pain after minimal trauma – sometimes a sneeze is all it needs

Infection (discitis and TB)

- Severe back pain in a systemically unwell patient with fever and night sweats
- Past history of TB may suggest Pott's disease

Inflammatory back pain (HLA-B27-associated conditions)

- Ankylosing spondylitis, psoriatic arthritis, enteropathic arthritis and reactive arthritis
- Typically, a young male of Caucasian origin
- Morning back stiffness lasting >1 hour which improves with exercise
- Reduced range of movement of spine with characteristic question mark posture in the late stages
- Patient usually feels more comfortable in a slightly stooped forward position

Non-spinal causes of back pain

- Dissecting aortic aneurysm – Sudden onset severe "tearing" back pain typically felt between the shoulder blades
- Ruptured abdominal aortic aneurysm – Sudden onset severe back/loin pain in someone aged >55 years; may have cardiovascular risk factors
- Fibromyalgia – More generalised aches and pains including arthralgia and myalgia
- Pancreatitis, endometriosis and renal calculi are rare causes of back pain

INVESTIGATIONS

- Back examination and lower limb neurological examination
- No further investigations if non-specific lower back pain
- FBC, CRP, ESR and autoimmune screen if inflammatory cause suspected
- Referral to neurosurgeons and MRI if radicular symptoms persist and are debilitating
- Referral to rheumatology for suspected inflammatory back pain
- Acute admission with MRI/CT scan if cord compression or cauda equina is suspected
- X-ray and a subsequent DEXA scan if a crush fracture is suspected

MANAGEMENT

- Advise to stay active and avoid prolonged bed rest
- Physiotherapy, regular analgesia and consider short-course muscle relaxants
- If disabling pain persists >1 year, consider referral to a pain specialist
- Cord compression – Dexamethasone and urgent surgery; radiotherapy in malignancy
- Cauda equina syndrome – Urgent surgery
- Ankylosing spondylitis – NSAIDs ± anti-TNF agents
- Osteoporosis – Bisphosphonates, vitamin D and calcium supplements

FURTHER READING

NICE CKS on back pain:
  Without radiculopathy, http://cks.nice.org.uk/back-pain-low-without-radiculopathy
  With radiculopathy, http://cks.nice.org.uk/sciatica-lumbar-radiculopathy

JOINT PAIN

INITIATING THE SESSION

- Greet the patient, ask an open question and screen for other problems

MEDICAL PERSPECTIVE

SEQUENCE OF EVENTS

- **Open question** – Can you tell me more about the pain you have been having?
- **Timeline** – How did the pain start? How has the pain progressed since then?

SYMPTOM ANALYSIS (SOCRATES)

- **Site** – Where is the pain?
- **Onset** – When did you first notice the pain? Was there any history of trauma?
- **Character** – What does the pain feel like?
- **Radiation** – Do you have pain anywhere else? (other joints)
- **Associated features** – *See systems review*
- **Timing** – When do you get the pain? Is it there all the time or does it come and go? Are the symptoms worse at any particular time of the day?
- **Exacerbating/relieving factors** – Does anything make it better? Does anything make it worse? Is it made better or worse by the cold? Is it made better or worse by exercise? Does resting the joint help the symptoms at all? What painkillers have you tried so far?
- **Severity** – If you had to rate the pain from 1 to 10 with 10 being the worst pain you can imagine, how would you score your pain?

SYSTEMS REVIEW

- **Stiffness** – Have you noticed any stiffness in your joint(s) when you wake up in the morning? How long does it last for?
- **Swelling** – Have you noticed any swelling, redness or heat in your joint(s)?
- **Infections** – Have you had any recent infections? Any sexually transmitted infections or gastroenteritis?
- **Uveitis/iritis** – Have you had painful or red eyes?
- **Spondyloarthropathy** – Have you had any back pain? Do you get any stiffness in your back in the morning? *If so,* for how long?
- **CTD** – Have you noticed any rashes anywhere on your body? Do you suffer from mouth ulcers? Dry eyes or mouth? Painfully cold hands that change colour?

> **RED FLAGS**
>
> *Early morning stiffness*
> *Improves with exercise*
> *Fever*
> *Known autoimmune*
> *   disorder*

PATIENT'S PERSPECTIVE

- **Feelings and effect on life** – How has your pain affected you day-to-day? Does it stop you doing things you used to be able to do? How about work?
- **Ideas** – What do you think is causing the pain?
- **Concerns** – Is there anything in particular you are concerned could be causing it? Is there anything in general that is concerning you about the pain?

- **Expectations** – When you made the appointment, other than getting my opinion, was there anything in particular you were hoping for?

BACKGROUND INFORMATION

PMH

- Do you suffer from any medical conditions?
- *Ask specifically about psoriasis, STIs, conjunctivitis and uveitis*
- Have you ever suffered from problems with your joint(s) in the past?

DH

- Do you take any medications?
- *Ask specifically about thiazides (could precipitate gout)*

FH

- Do any conditions run in your family?
- Does anyone suffer from inflammatory arthritis such as rheumatoid arthritis?

SH

- Are you working presently? *If so,* what is your job? What does that involve?
- Can you tell me about your home situation (*occupants and any difficulties*)?
- Has your problem affected your job or home life in any way?
- Do you smoke? How many cigarettes do you smoke a day? For how long?
- Do you drink alcohol? How much do you drink in a week?

CLOSING THE SESSION

- summary ± examination/explanation and planning/contract

> **IMPORTANT POINTS**
>
> - Stiffness that improves with exercise, swelling and heat are important features that indicate an inflammatory cause
> - Many arthritides are associated with systemic symptoms. Extra-articular features may provide useful clues as to the underlying pathology
> - The pattern of joints involved gives a good idea about the likely underlying condition. Is it small or large joint; symmetrical or asymmetrical; monoarthritis, oligoarthritis or polyarthritis?
> - Beware the acutely hot and swollen joint. Always consider septic arthritis

DIFFERENTIAL DIAGNOSIS

It is vital to identify patients with a likely underlying inflammatory arthritis quickly in order to allow prompt referral and early and aggressive disease management as it has been shown that this affects the prognosis in inflammatory arthritides.

INFLAMMATORY CONDITIONS

RHEUMATOID ARTHRITIS

- Symmetrical polyarthritis that typically causes synovitis in small joints, particularly the hands and feet, although large joints can also be affected
- Morning stiffness lasting >1 hour, along with pain that improves with exercise
- Increased risk of CVD, osteoporosis, scleritis and interstitial lung disease

SERONEGATIVE SPONDYLOARTHRITIS (HLA-B27-associated conditions)

- Psoriatic arthritis, ankylosing spondylitis, enteropathic arthritis and reactive arthritis
- Typically, there is an asymmetrical oligoarthritis affecting large joints – the spine is frequently involved with sacroileitis most commonly – and enthesitis
- Morning stiffness lasting >1 hour, along with pain that improves with exercise
- Particularly consider in a history of psoriasis/bowel disorders/recent infection

SYSTEMIC LUPUS ERYTHEMATOSUS

- Arthralgia and/or symmetrical small joint polyarthritis (non-erosive)
- Typically affects non-Caucasian females with age of onset in early adulthood
- Common features include oral ulcers, Raynaud's phenomenon, dry eyes and/or mouth, photosensitivity, malar rash, discoid rash, fever and general malaise

NON-INFLAMMATORY CONDITIONS

OSTEOARTHRITIS

- Pain in older patients that is worse with exercise and at least partially relieved by rest
- Symmetrical oligo- or polyarthritis that most frequently affects hips, knees and hands
- History of previous injury to the joint and/or obesity (especially for knee OA)

GOUT

- Joint pain, oedema and erythema that develops acutely (classically overnight)
- Usually it is a large joint monoarthritis affecting the first metatarsophalangeal joint, but it can affect any joint and can be polyarticular
- History of excessive alcohol and red meat consumption, hypertension, renal failure, diuretics and being male!

FIBROMYALGIA

- Myalgia that can be reproduced over specific trigger points without joint involvement
- Patient may complain of swelling despite objectively no swelling being present
- Associated with depression and irritable bowel syndrome

SEPTIC ARTHRITIS

- An acutely hot, very painful and swollen joint in an unwell patient with fever
- There may be a history of immunosuppression and/or trauma
- Unilateral swollen joint with local tenderness and preceding history of injury

INVESTIGATIONS

- Examine joint(s) in question and screen other joints; look for evidence of extra-articular features such as rash, nail changes, gouty tophi, lung fibrosis
- Bloods – FBC, U&Es, LFTs, CRP and ESR
- Rheumatoid factor and anti-CCP for RA; autoimmune screen if suspecting CTD
- Blood cultures and synovial fluid analysis if suspecting septic arthritis
- Serum urate if suspecting gout (NB: may be falsely low in acute attacks)
- X-rays of joint(s) for evidence of erosive disease (usually of hands and feet)

MANAGEMENT

- Physiotherapy has a role in each chronic condition
- Osteoarthritis – Exercise, weight loss, paracetamol and/or topical anti-inflammatory
- Rheumatoid arthritis – Early DMARDs (e.g. methotrexate); anti-TNF therapy if conventional DMARDs fail
- Gout – Treat acute attack with NSAIDs; after acute episode resolves, review precipitating factors and consider allopurinol for long-term prevention
- Seronegative spondyloarthritis – NSAIDs, DMARDS in peripheral arthritis and anti-TNF therapy
- SLE – Hydroxychloroquine for mild symptoms; steroids and DMARDs for joint disease; high-dose steroids and potent immunosuppressants for end-organ disease
- Fibromyalgia – Patient education; amitriptyline currently first-line medication
- Septic arthritis – Broad spectrum IV antibiotics; washout in theatre

FURTHER READING

Arthritis Research UK guidance on approaching the patient with joint pain, http://www.arthritisresearchuk.org/health-professionals-and-students/reports/hands-on/hands-on-autumn-2012.aspx

NICE CKS on:
Knee pain, http://cks.nice.org.uk/knee-pain-assessment
Osteoarthritis, http://cks.nice.org.uk/osteoarthritis
Rheumatoid arthritis, http://cks.nice.org.uk/rheumatoid-arthritis

Surgery

6

ABDOMINAL PAIN

INITIATING THE SESSION

- Greet the patient, ask an open question and screen for other problems

MEDICAL PERSPECTIVE

SEQUENCE OF EVENTS

- **Open question** – Can you tell me more about the pain you have been having?
- **Timeline** – How did the pain start? How has the pain progressed since then?

SYMPTOM ANALYSIS (SOCRATES)

- **Site** – Where exactly do you get this pain? Can you point to it precisely? Where did the pain first manifest – has it moved?
- **Onset** – How long ago did this pain start? *Minutes, hours, days, weeks, months?*
- **Character** – What does the pain feel like?
- **Radiation** – Does the pain move anywhere else? Can you show me? Does it go into your back/around the side/groin/testicles? Do you get shoulder tip pain?
- **Associated features** – *See systems review*
- **Timing** – Is the pain there all the time or does it come and go? How long does it last for? How long do you get between episodes of pain? Is there any particular time when you have noticed you get the pain (*day, night, mealtimes, menses*)?
- **Exacerbating/relieving factors** – What, if anything, brings the pain on? Does anything make it better or worse? Have you taken anything to relieve the pain? Is it getting better/worse with time? Does body position make a difference?
- **Severity** – If you had to rate the pain from 1 to 10 with 10 being the worst pain you can imagine, how would you score this pain now? How would it score it at its worst?

RED FLAGS

Acute pain
Chronic night-time pain
Unexplained weight loss
Dysphagia
Haematemesis/melaena
Change in bowel habit
Bleeding per rectum
Haematuria
Risk factors for ACS

SYSTEMS REVIEW

- **GIT** – Have you had any difficulty swallowing? Any heartburn or indigestion? Any vomiting? *If so,* have you noticed any blood in the vomitus? Any change in your bowel motions? Any blood or mucus in your stools?
- **GUT** – How have your waterworks been? Have you noticed any blood in the urine? Any pain when passing urine? Are you passing urine more frequently? How have your periods been (*if relevant*)? *Date of last menstrual period + cycle*
- **CVS** – Do you ever get chest pain? Does this pain come on during exercise?
- **Constitutional** – Have you noticed any weight loss? How has your appetite been? Have you felt feverish?

PATIENT'S PERSPECTIVE

- **Feelings and effect on life** – How has the pain affected your daily life?
- **Ideas** – What do you think is causing the pain?
- **Concerns** – Is there anything in particular you are concerned could be causing it? Is there anything in general that is concerning you about the pain?
- **Expectations** – When you made the appointment, other than getting my opinion, was there anything in particular you were hoping for?

BACKGROUND INFORMATION

PMH

- Do you suffer from any medical conditions? Have you ever had this pain before?

DH

- Are you currently taking any medications? Do you have any allergies?
- *Ask specifically about steroids and NSAIDs*

FH

- Do any conditions run in the family?
- Has anyone else in your family suffered from this kind of pain? Were they diagnosed?

SH

- Do you drink alcohol? How much do you drink in a week?
- Do you smoke?
- Are you working presently? *If so,* what is your job? What does that involve?
- Can you tell me about your home situation (*occupants and any difficulties*)?
- Has your problem affected your job or home life in any way?

CLOSING THE SESSION

- summary ± examination/explanation and planning/contract

- After taking a history of the pain you must consider differentials in your mind and ask relevant questions about the systems involved
- Never forget that ACS can present as abdominal pain and as such relevant questions must be asked to rule this out

DIFFERENTIAL DIAGNOSIS

The commonest causes of abdominal pain are:

- Constipation – often mimicking sub-acute obstruction
- Menstrual pain
- Appendicitis – commonest cause of an acute abdomen presenting to A&E
- UTI – one of the commonest organic causes of abdominal pain in primary care
- Irritable bowel syndrome – a diagnosis of exclusion
- Non-specific pain

It is valuable to divide abdominal pain into acute versus chronic conditions and consider the most likely diagnoses that may present with pain in that area.

The pathophysiology of abdominal pain may be divided into parietal, visceral and referred. Parietal or somatic pain is well localised and is caused by local inflammation and is a consequence of infection, irritation etc. Visceral pain is usually due to distension of a viscus and is poorly localised. Upper abdominal pain usually reflects stomach, duodenal, gallbladder, liver or pancreas pathology; central abdominal pain reflects those areas supplied by the superior mesenteric artery i.e. small bowel, appendix and proximal colon; lower abdominal pain reflects pathology in the lower colon and genito-urinary tract. Referred pain is usually secondary to cardiopulmonary conditions but may also be secondary to abdominal wall problems such as herpes zoster or muscle haematoma.

ACUTE ABDOMINAL PAIN

Acute abdominal pain almost always has a definitive pathophysiology, and it is this group that requires the most attention in terms of urgent diagnosis. Amongst the diagnoses behind acute abdominal pain, several diagnoses require immediate management. These include ruptured aortic aneurysm, torsion of the testis, ectopic pregnancy, spontaneous intra-abdominal haemorrhage, acute mesenteric ischaemia and strangulated bowel. All of these have a vascular compromise. Most other acute abdominal conditions benefit from a period of stabilisation before definitive management.

CHRONIC ABDOMINAL PAIN

Chronic abdominal pain is pain that has been present for more than 6 months. There is a multitude of possible causes. Essentially, they may be divided into organic and functional aetiology. Up to 25% of the normal adult population will have chronic abdominal pain.

INVESTIGATIONS

ACUTE ABDOMINAL PAIN

- Bloods – FBC, U&Es, LFTs, amylase and glucose
- Urinalysis
- Pregnancy test (*where relevant*)
- Radiological assessment (*see below*)

A FAST (focussed assessment with sonography for trauma) scan in A&E can pick up aortic aneurysm, ruptured spleen and ruptured ectopic pregnancy. The most valuable investigation to inform diagnosis is a CT or MR scan. It is important to remember however that the result of any investigation should be taken in the context of the obtained history and subsequent examination. E.g. there is a false negative rate of at least 10% in CT scans.

CHRONIC ABDOMINAL PAIN

- Bloods and urinalysis
- *H. pylori* stool antigen test (dyspepsia)
- Faecal calprotectin (detects neutrophils in GIT; useful in suspected IBD)
- Endoscopy (upper and/or lower GIT)
- Ultrasound scan to look for gallstones and urogynaecological pathology
- CT or MR abdomen (this tends to be directed by secondary care rather than GP)

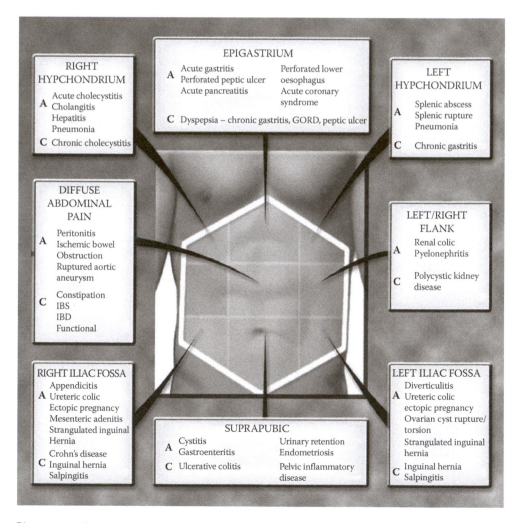

Diagram showing causes of acute and chronic abdominal pain by site

FURTHER READING

BMJ best practice article on acute abdominal pain, http://bestpractice.bmj.com/best-practice/monograph/503.html
Patient.co.uk professional article on the acute abdomen, http://patient.info/doctor/acute-abdomen
NICE CKS on dyspepsia, http://cks.nice.org.uk/dyspepsia-unidentified-cause

BLEEDING PER RECTUM

INITIATING THE SESSION

- Greet the patient, ask an open question and screen for other problems

MEDICAL PERSPECTIVE

SEQUENCE OF EVENTS

- **Open question** – Can you tell me more about this bleeding?
- **Timeline** – How did it start? How has it progressed since then?

SYMPTOM ANALYSIS (SOCRATES)

- **Site** – Can I just clarify the bleeding is coming from the back passage, not the front?
- **Onset** – When did you first notice this?
- **Character/colour** – What colour is the blood? Fresh red? Dark? How much blood have you noticed? Streaks? Teaspoon? More?
- **Radiation (to paper/pan)** – Did you notice the blood in the pan or on the tissue paper? Is it mixed in with the stool?
- **Associated features** – *See systems review*
- **Timing** – Has this happened before?
- **Exacerbating factors** – Does anything bring it on, such as episodes of constipation? Any recent trauma to the area?
- **Smell** (melaena) – Have you noticed it to be particularly foul smelling, dark or tarry?

SYSTEMS REVIEW

- **Pain** – Have you had any pain in your abdomen?
- **Lower GIT** – What are your stools like? Any mucus? How often are you passing stools? Is this normal for you? Have you noticed any itching around the back passage? Have you been nauseous or sick? Have you vomited up any blood?
- **IBD** – Have you had any mouth ulcers? Fever? Painful red eye? Joint or back pain?
- **Foreign travel** – Have you been abroad recently? *If so,* where?
- **Constitutional** – Have you been feeling more tired than normal recently? Have you noticed any unintentional weight loss? How has your appetite been?

PATIENT'S PERSPECTIVE

- **Feelings and effect on life** – Have your symptoms had any effect on your daily life?
- **Ideas** – What do you think is causing the bleeding?
- **Concerns** – Some people think of cancer when they get bleeding from the back passage. Are you concerned about that? Is there anything else that is concerning you?
- **Expectations** – Would I be right in thinking you made the appointment to check if it was anything serious? Was there anything in particular you were hoping for?

BACKGROUND INFORMATION

PMH

- Do you suffer from any medical conditions? *"PRHIM"*:
    - **P**eptic ulcers
    - **R**ecent GIT surgery
    - **H**aemorrhoids
    - **I**BD and diverticulitis
    - **M**alignancy

DH

- Do you take any regular medications? Any over-the-counter medications?

FH

- Do any conditions run in the family?
- *Ask about IBD and malignancy (colorectal and ovarian carcinoma – and determine which relatives they were and what age they were when they were diagnosed)*

SH

- Do you smoke? How many cigarettes do you smoke a day? For how long?
- Do you drink alcohol? How much do you drink in a week?
- Are you working presently? *If so,* what is your job? What does that involve?
- Can you tell me about your home situation (*occupants and any difficulties*)?
- Has your problem affected your job or home life in any way?

CLOSING THE SESSION

- summary ± examination/explanation and planning/contract

IMPORTANT POINTS

- Bleeding of any nature can be particularly frightening and/or embarrassing for most patients and therefore it is important to approach this history in a sympathetic manner – if the patient is tentative, initially help put their mind at ease e.g. "Some people are frightened or embarrassed to talk about these problems, but it is a common issue and it is important that it is explored so thank you for coming in today"
- Never forget to ask about other red flag symptoms (e.g. cachexia, persistent change in bowel habit for 6 weeks or more, anaemia and upper GIT symptoms)
- Family history is very important here – do not forget!
- The colour of the blood and extent it is mixed in with the stool can help determine where the bleed is likely to originate from. PR bleeding from the upper GIT is partially digested, producing melaena – a dark extremely foul-smelling stool; bleeds of anorectal pathology will be fresh red and those in between are usually darker and mixed in with the stool
- In lesions affecting the caecum/ascending colon, there may be no change in bowel habit as faecal matter in this part of the colon is liquid/semi-solid (hence, unexplained anaemia must be investigated), whereas lesions in the sigmoid colon/rectum will often cause a change in bowel habit due to obstruction

DIFFERENTIAL DIAGNOSIS

HAEMORRHOIDS (MOST COMMON)

- Fresh red blood on the toilet paper or in the pan
- Associated with pruritus ani, but not usually painful
- History of constipation and straining

COLORECTAL CANCER (MOST SERIOUS)

- Age over 55 years (unless familial predisposition mentioned)
- Red flag symptoms include cachexia, rectal bleeding, abdominal mass found and change in bowel habit lasting 6 weeks or more
- Always consider in men of any age or non-menstruating women with unexplained iron-deficiency anaemia
- Previous history of malignancy, IBD and coeliac disease

ANAL FISSURE

- Fresh red blood seen in the toilet paper, not the pan
- Can be acute or chronic with pruritus ani commonly also found
- Fissures may cause severe pain during defecation, deterring the patient from regularly opening their bowels, causing constipation which exacerbates the problem

GASTROENTERITIS

- Recent history of eating uncooked/poorly prepared food and/or foreign travel
- Diarrhoea (may be watery, bloody or simply loose) and vomiting
- Household members/contacts may also be unwell with similar symptoms

DIVERTICULAR DISEASE

- Middle-age/elderly patients with bloody diarrhoea and pain in left iliac fossa
- Can lead to diverticulitis, with fever, nausea and vomiting
- Risk factors include obesity and low dietary fibre

INFLAMMATORY BOWEL DISEASE

- Diarrhoea with blood and mucus, and lower abdominal pain
- Night-time pain and weight loss in younger patients are red flags for IBD
- Bleeding per rectum more commonly occurs in ulcerative colitis than Crohn's disease

ANGIODYSPLASIA

- Painless bleeding due to enlarged friable blood vessels in colon
- Can be bright red, dark blood mixed in with faeces or even present as melaena
- Usually occurs in elderly patients

UPPER GI BLEED

- Large volume bleed, unwell patient that may be haemodynamically shocked
- Dark tarry stool produced (melaena)
- Haematemesis and other red flag symptoms may be present
- Previous history of dyspepsia, peptic ulcers, chronic liver disease and/or long-term anti-inflammatory use

INVESTIGATIONS

- Full abdominal examination, including PR examination
- Bloods – FBC, U&Es, LFT, clotting, CRP, group and save or cross-match (if severe)
- Stool culture if associated with diarrhoea
- Faecal calprotectin if IBD suspected
- Sigmoidoscopy/colonoscopy ± upper GIT endoscopy
- Staging CT abdomen/pelvis if malignancy suspected on endoscopy

MANAGEMENT

- Give advice on diet and lifestyle to help with constipation (including fluid intake)
- Laxatives for constipation exacerbating anorectal and diverticular disease
- Anal fissure – Measures to avoid constipation; short course of topical local anaesthetic or steroid cream; GTN ointment and/or surgery in chronic cases
- Haemorrhoids – Measures to avoid constipation; rubber band ligation; sclerosant therapy; haemorrhoidectomy
- Angiodysplasia – Ensure patient is haemodynamically stable first; endoscopic obliteration; surgical resection in isolated refractive cases
- 2-week referral for patients with red flag symptoms
- Ulcerative colitis – Sulfasalazine; pancolectomy; steroids for flare-ups
- Gastroenteritis – Rehydration; antibiotics only if indicated by stool culture
- Diverticular disease – High-fibre diet and bulk-producing laxatives if no better

FURTHER READING

Royal College of Surgeons guidance on management of rectal bleeding, https://www.rcseng.ac.uk/healthcare-bodies/docs/published-guides/rectal-bleeding

NICE CKS on haemorrhoids, http://cks.nice.org.uk/haemorrhoids

LUMPS, BUMPS AND SWELLINGS

NB: *There is a separate history on neck lumps, pp. 125*

INITIATING THE SESSION

- Greet the patient, ask an open question and screen for other problems

MEDICAL PERSPECTIVE

SEQUENCE OF EVENTS

- **Open question** – I understand that you have noticed a lump. Would you like to tell me about it?
- **Timeline** – How did it start? How long ago did you first notice the lump (*Days, weeks, months*)? How has it progressed since then? Is it getting bigger or smaller? Is it there all the time or does it come and go? Have you ever had this lump/a similar lump before? *If so,* what happened?

SYMPTOM ANALYSIS

- **Site** – Where exactly is the lump? Can you point to it precisely?
- **Pain** – Is it painful? Does it interfere with doing things?
- **Trigger** – Does anything make the lump more noticeable e.g. change in posture?
- **Other lumps** – Are there any other similar lumps that you have noticed?

SYSTEMS REVIEW

RED FLAGS

Weight loss
Hard, irregular lump
Progressively enlarging
Red flags in systems reviewed

NB: A relevant systems review here is dependent upon the site and nature of the lump seen.

PATIENT'S PERSPECTIVE

- **Feelings and effect on life** – Has your lump had any effect on your daily life?
- **Ideas** – What do you think is causing the lump?
- **Concerns** – Some people think of cancer when they get notice lumps. Are you concerned about that? Is there anything else that is concerning you?
- **Expectations** – Would I be right in thinking you made the appointment to check if it was anything serious? Was there anything in particular you were hoping for?

BACKGROUND INFORMATION

PMH

- Do you suffer from any medical conditions?
- *Abdominal lumps/swelling* – Previous surgery (e.g. incisional hernias)
- *Limb lumps/swelling* – Rheumatoid arthritis; osteoarthritis; varicose veins

DH

- Are you taking any medications? Do you have any allergies?

FH

- Do any condition run in the family? (*e.g. lipomatosis, neurofibromatosis*)
- Has anyone else in your family suffered from similar problems?

SH

- Do you smoke? How many cigarettes do you smoke a day? For how long?
- Do you drink alcohol? How much do you drink in a week?
- Are you working presently? *If so,* what is your job? What does that involve?
- Can you tell me about your home situation (*occupants and any difficulties*)?
- Has your problem affected your job or home life in any way?
- Has anyone at home or at work been ill with anything recently? *If so, specify*

CLOSING THE SESSION

- summary ± examination/explanation and planning/contract

IMPORTANT POINTS

- This is likely to be a combined history and examination station, in which most of the time will be spent on the examination aspect. If given sufficient time for a history, you may wish to enquire about every aspect of the history, but in most cases it will suffice to ask about the characteristics of the lump
- Always consider whether the lump could represent a malignancy and ask relevant questions to help determine the likelihood of this (e.g. weight loss, non-tender, previous cancer, heavy smoking history etc.)
- Typical symptoms in OSCEs include neck lumps, abdominal swellings/masses such as hernias (commonly inguinal or incisional), polycystic kidney disease (renal mass), simple lumps such as lipomas, chronic conditions such as neurofibromatosis etc.

DIFFERENTIAL DIAGNOSIS

It is impossible to encompass here a complete differential diagnosis for lumps (which could be anywhere and almost anything) prior to a specific examination; however, in the context of an OSCE and where there is a real-life patient, the diagnoses listed below are perhaps the more common presentations.

Neck – *See neck lump history, pp. 125*

ABDOMEN

- Inguinal hernia
- Incisional hernia

- Para/umbilical hernia
- Polycystic kidney disease

LIMBS

- Arteriovenous fistula in dialysis patients
- Joint effusion
- Ganglion

ANYWHERE

- Lipoma
- Cyst (e.g. sebaceous)
- Lymph node
- Neurofibroma

INVESTIGATIONS AND MANAGEMENT

It is important to remember that the result of any investigation must be considered in the light of the obtained history and subsequent examination. Therefore, the investigation of a lump ranges from doing nothing (a simple lipoma) to detailed cytology following fine-needle aspiration (many neck lumps).

Likewise, the management of a lump depends on the clinical scenario. Not all lumps need to be removed and clinical acumen must be used.

FURTHER READING

NICE CKS on breast cancer recognition and referral, http://cks.nice.org.uk/breast-cancer-recognition-and-referral

WEIGHT LOSS

INITIATING THE SESSION

- Greet the patient, ask an open question and screen for other problems

MEDICAL PERSPECTIVE

SEQUENCE OF EVENTS

- **Open question** – Can you tell me more about this bleeding?
- **Timeline** – How did it start? How has it progressed since then? Over what period of time has this occurred?

SYMPTOM ANALYSIS

- **Amount** – How much weight have you lost? Have you actually weighed yourself?
- **Patient's ideas** – What do you think could be causing the weight loss?
- **Intention** – Was this weight loss intentional or not?
- **Appetite** – How has your appetite been? Have you been eating normally?
- **Exercise** – Have you been exercising more than usual?
- **Constitutional** – Have you had any episodes of fever or sweating, especially at night?

SYSTEMS REVIEW

- **RS** – Have you noticed a cough recently? *If so,* do you bring anything up? Any blood? Have you found yourself more breathless than previously?
- **GIT** – Have you had any difficulty swallowing? Any pain in your tummy? Any heartburn? Any vomiting? *If so,* have you noticed any blood in the vomitus? Any change in your bowel motions? Any blood in your stools?
- **GUT** – How are your waterworks? Have you noticed any blood in the urine? Any pain when passing urine? Are you going more frequently? How have your periods been (*if relevant*)? *Any postcoital, intermenstrual or postmenopausal bleeding?*
- **NS** – Have you had any weakness in any of your muscles? Any pins and needles or strange sensations? Any headaches? Any problems with your vision or other senses?
- **MS** – Do you have pain in your muscles, bones or joints? Are they stiff in the mornings?
- **ENT** – Have you had a persistent sore throat? A hoarse voice? Any neck lumps?

> **RED FLAGS**
>
> *Unintentional weight loss*
> *Red flags in systems reviewed*

PATIENT'S PERSPECTIVE

- **Feelings and effect on life** – What effect has all this had on your daily life?
- **Ideas** – What do you think is causing the weight loss?
- **Concerns** – Is there anything in particular you are concerned could be causing the weight loss? Is there anything in general that is concerning you?
- **Expectations** – Would I be right in thinking you made the appointment to check if it was anything serious? Was there anything in particular you were hoping for?

BACKGROUND INFORMATION

PMH

- Do you suffer from any medical conditions?
- *Ask about recent illness, thyrotoxicosis, chronic infections, IBD and previous cancer*

DH

- Are you taking any medications? Have any been changed recently? Any allergies?

FH

- Do any specific conditions run in your family? Are there any specific cancers that are common in your family? *If so, take history of relation and age at diagnosis*

SH

- How much alcohol do you drink?
- Do you smoke? How many do/did you smoke a day? For how long?
- Are you working presently? *If so,* what is your job? What does that involve?
- Can you tell me about your home situation (*occupants and any difficulties*)? Who cooks for you? What do you eat in a standard day?
- Has your problem affected your job or home life in any way?

CLOSING THE SESSION

- summary ± examination/explanation and planning/contract

IMPORTANT POINTS

- In other histories when asking about weight loss, if the patient is unsure about weight loss it can be useful asking about clothes which no longer fit or if they have had to start using a belt for their trousers
- A good systems review is key to this history, as the presenting complaint can be attributed to many different systems
- Try to estimate how much weight has been lost and if it has been recent
- Ask when the patients actually last weighed themselves to gain an idea of reliability

DIFFERENTIAL DIAGNOSIS

Weight loss is due to either inadequate intake, malabsorption, reduced anabolism, increased catabolism or a combination. Essentially, if calories used up are greater than intake, then weight loss will occur. Increased catabolism is common in acute and chronic infections but is seen in malignancy, inflammatory conditions, post-surgery. Surgical sieves (e.g. CANDITIME – below) can be useful ways of reciting causes of any given condition. Weight loss may represent the first manifestation of a potentially serious condition or be nothing more than an external manifestation of anxiety or depression.

CONGENITAL (FAILURE TO THRIVE)

- Genetic or chromosomal abnormalities e.g. Down's syndrome and cystic fibrosis
- Constitutional
- Others (*see failure to thrive history pp. 183*)

ACQUIRED

NEOPLASM

- Primary or secondary malignancy

DEGENERATIVE

- COPD
- Multiple sclerosis

INFECTION/INFLAMMATORY

- Viral – Short coryzal illness or more chronic infection (e.g. CMV, EBV or HIV)
- Bacterial (e.g. streptococcal pneumonia) or fungal (e.g. cryptococcal pneumonia)
- Other infection (e.g. TB)
- Inflammatory conditions – CTD (e.g. SLE), RA, IBD or vasculitis

TRAUMA (LESS LIKELY CAUSE FOR WEIGHT LOSS)

Iatrogenic/Idiopathic

- Recent major surgery (e.g. gastrectomy)

Miscellaneous

- Anorexia nervosa
- Depression and/or other psychiatric diagnoses

Endocrine

- Hyperthyroidism

INVESTIGATIONS

- Physical examination of all systems
- Bloods – FBC, U&Es, LFTs, glucose, TFTs, CRP and ESR
- Urinalysis
- Chest x-ray
- CT scan (area depending upon clinical suspicion)

The investigation of weight loss is difficult as the potential causes are multiple. The above is a rough guide, but clinical judgement is important to fine-tune this list further.

FURTHER READING

NICE guidelines on:
Cancer recognition and referral, https://www.nice.org.uk/guidance/NG12
Malnutrition, https://www.nice.org.uk/Guidance/CG32

INTERMITTENT CLAUDICATION

INITIATING THE SESSION

- Greet the patient, ask an open question and screen for other problems

MEDICAL PERSPECTIVE

SEQUENCE OF EVENTS

- **Open question** – Can you tell me more about this pain/cramping sensation?
- **Timeline** – How did it start? How has it progressed since then? Over what period of time has this occurred?

SYMPTOM ANALYSIS (SOCRATES)

- **Site** – Where do you get the pain? (*buttock, thigh, calf*)
- **Onset** – Did it come on suddenly or gradually?
- **Character** – What does it feel like? (*cramping, tightening of muscles*)
- **Radiation** – Does the pain go anywhere else?
- **Associated factors** – Do you get any pain at night? Have you noticed any ulcers in your legs or feet? *If so,* are they painful?
- **Timing** – Do you get the pain when walking or at rest? Any previous episodes and interventions?
- **Exacerbating and relieving factors** – Is it relieved by rest? Is it made worse if you walk faster or up a hill? Does cold weather affect it?
- **Severity** – How badly does it affect you? How far can you walk before stopping? Do you want to have something done about it?

RED FLAGS

Rest pain
Arterial ulcers
Tissue loss/amputations
Smoking

PATIENT'S PERSPECTIVE

- **Feelings and effect on life** – What effect has the pain had on your daily life?
- **Ideas** – What do you think is causing the pain?
- **Concerns** – Is there anything in particular you are concerned could be causing the pain? Is there anything in general that is concerning you?
- **Expectations** – Was there anything in particular you were hoping for when you made the appointment to see me today?

BACKGROUND INFORMATION

PMH

- Do you suffer from any medical conditions? Have you had any previous surgery?
- *Ask about diabetes, previous stroke, ACS, hypertension and hypercholesterolaemia*

DH

- Are you taking any medications? Do you have any allergies?

FH

- Do any conditions run in the family?

SH

- Do you smoke? (*Have you ever smoked/quantify*)
- Do you drink alcohol? How much do you drink?
- Are you still in work/employed? *If so*, what is your job? What does that involve?
- Can you tell me about your home situation (*occupants and any difficulties*)?
- Has your problem affected your job or home life in any way?

CLOSING THE SESSION

- summary ± examination/explanation and planning/contract

> **IMPORTANT POINTS**
>
> - Claudication pain does not occur at rest, sitting or lying down – check that the patient never gets this particular pain except when walking
> - Older patients may have other exercise-limiting conditions, such as dyspnoea, so be certain to establish which the more significant problem is for them
> - Use medications as a way of cross-checking the patient's past medical history (they will often forget to mention hypertension as they consider this to be under control!)

DIFFERENTIAL DIAGNOSIS

PERIPHERAL VASCULAR DISEASE

- Claudication pain is a cramping pain in the calf, thigh or buttocks
- Brought on reproducibly by exercise and relieved by rest (patients often pretend to "window shop" until the pain disappears)
- Exacerbated by walking faster or up hills and also by cold weather
- Risk factors/associated factors for atherosclerosis:
  - Smoking
  - Diabetes
  - Hypercholesterolaemia
  - Ischaemic heart disease and stroke
  - Hypertension
  - Family history
  - Male sex
- Rest pain may indicate critical limb ischaemia

OSTEOARTHRITIS

- Pain localised to feet, ankles or knees (i.e. joints)
- Often pain elsewhere e.g. hands and neck
- Very common; often co-exists with claudication
- Not brought on by walking a certain distance as is usually the case with claudication

SCIATICA

- Shooting pain down the back of a leg to the feet
- History of lower back pain

SPINAL CLAUDICATION

- Often relieved when walking up a hill
- Often has associated limb numbness
- Relatively uncommon

DEEP VEIN THROMBOSIS

- Tender, swollen, warm and red leg
- Risk factors: immobilisation, pregnancy, cancer, combined oral contraceptive pill, family history, clotting disorders

MUSCULOSKELETAL INJURY

- History of preceding injury
- Localised pain and tenderness

INVESTIGATIONS

- Full peripheral, vascular, cardiovascular and neurological examination
- Bloods – U&Es, fasting glucose or HbA1c, cholesterol (HDL/LDL)
- Blood pressure – Both arms (asymptomatic subclavian artery occlusion is quite common and will give a low blood pressure)
- Ankle brachial pressure indices (Doppler derived)
- Duplex scan of common femoral and superficial femoral arteries

MANAGEMENT

- Stop smoking – Firm counselling is needed with the emphasis on taking responsibility for their health; complete cessation is the aim
- Exercise (walking), including supervised exercise programmes if available
- Point out alternative ways of getting from A to B (bus, cycling, car etc.)
- Start secondary risk prevention measures (e.g. clopidogrel, statin)
- Consider a trial of conservative management and review in 6 months
- Consider prescribing naftidrofuryl oxalate if exercise has not helped and the patient does not wish to have surgical intervention (stop if no benefit after 3–6 months)
- If intervention (e.g. angioplasty or bypass graft) is considered, then an angiogram is required. Be aware of risk of metformin and contrast media (possible renal failure)

FURTHER READING

NICE CKS on peripheral vascular disease, http://cks.nice.org.uk/peripheral-arterial-disease

Urology/renal medicine

HAEMATURIA

INITIATING THE SESSION

- Greet the patient, ask an open question and screen for other problems

MEDICAL PERSPECTIVE

SEQUENCE OF EVENTS

- **Open question** – Can you tell me more about what you have noticed?
- **Timeline** – How did it start? How has it progressed since then? Over what period of time has this occurred?

SYMPTOM ANALYSIS

- **Clarify site** – When do you notice the blood? Is it only when you pass urine? Is there any chance it could be coming from elsewhere?
- **Colour** – What colour is your urine? Have you recently eaten any beetroot?
- **Timing** – Is there always blood in your urine or does it come and go? Have you had this before? Is the blood present at the start of urination, the end or throughout?
- **Severity** – Do you pass any clots in your urine?

SYSTEMS REVIEW

- **Abdominal pain** – Do you have pain in your abdomen or back?
- **Dysuria** – Do you have any pain when you pass urine?
- **Frequency/urgency** – Do you find yourself needing to go to the toilet to pass urine more often? Do you get sudden irrepressible urges to pass water?
- **Obstruction** – Do you have difficulty getting the stream started? Is there prolonged dribbling at the end? Is your stream powerful or weak? How often do you get up at night to pass urine?

> **RED FLAGS**
>
> Weight loss
> Painless haematuria
> Trauma
> Smoking
> Work in dye factory

- **Constitutional** – Have you been unwell or feverish recently? How is your appetite? Have you lost any weight? Have you gained much weight? Do your ankles swell?
- **Glomerulonephritides** – Have you had a sore throat recently? Have you noticed any rashes or sore joints?
- **Pulmonary-renal conditions** – Have you recently coughed up any blood?
- **Trauma** – Have you had any trauma to your stomach or groin recently?

PATIENT'S PERSPECTIVE

- **Feelings and effect on life** – Have your symptoms had any effect on your daily life?
- **Ideas** – What do you think is causing the blood in your urine?
- **Concerns** – Is there anything in particular you are concerned could be causing it? Is there anything in general that is concerning you?
- **Expectations** – Did you just come to check whether it might be serious? Or was there something in particular you had in mind for today?

BACKGROUND INFORMATION

PMH

- Do you suffer from any medical conditions?
- *Ask about renal disease, previous UTIs and prostate/renal/bladder cancer*

DH

- Do you take any regular medications? Do you have any allergies?

FH

- Do any conditions run in the family?
- *Ask about renal disease (including polycystic kidney disease) and bleeding disorders*
- Does anyone else in the family have blood in their urine? *Asymptomatic haematuria can be benign and familial*

SH

- Do you smoke? How many do you smoke a day? For how long?
- Are you working presently? *If so,* what is your job? What does that involve? Have you ever worked with industrial chemicals or dyes?
- Can you tell me about your home situation (*occupants and any difficulties*)?
- Has your problem affected your job or home life in any way?

CLOSING THE SESSION

- summary ± examination/explanation and planning/contract

DIFFERENTIAL DIAGNOSIS

Haematuria can be frank or microscopic. The causes of these are generally quite different. Frank haematuria is more likely due to a lower urinary tract lesion, whereas microscopic haematuria is suggestive of glomerular disease. This is not a perfect rule however. Frank haematuria has a 20–25% chance of being due to malignancy which is why it is much more aggressively investigated than microscopic haematuria. Microscopic haematuria is relatively more common and should only be considered pathological when recurring or associated with lower urinary tract symptoms.

MALIGNANCY

RENAL CELL CARCINOMA

- Triad of flank pain, haematuria and an abdominal mass (late presentation)
- Can be found incidentally on examination in patients with hypertension or anaemia
- Constitutional symptoms of weight loss, fever and fatigue
- May present with paraneoplastic syndrome causing excessive renin, parathyroid hormone or erythropoietin

TRANSITIONAL CELL CARCINOMA

- Painless, intermittent haematuria in older males is a worrying sign
- Can affect the ureters or urethra, but most commonly affects the bladder
- The classical association is working with industrial dyes, but nowadays smoking is by far the biggest risk factor in the UK
- Schistosomiasis is the biggest cause of bladder cancer elsewhere (e.g. Africa)

RENAL CALCULI

- Acute onset of excruciating flank/abdominal pain, radiating from "loin to groin," with associated nausea and vomiting
- Pain in renal colic is more constant than in biliary/intestinal colic, but often there are periods of relief in which the patient has a dull ache
- Often however calculi are asymptomatic and found incidentally on imaging
- Typically affects men in their 30s to 50s

URINARY TRACT INFECTION

- Cystitis typically produces urinary frequency, urgency and dysuria
- Fever, suprapubic pain and urethral discharge may also be present
- The urine may be cloudy with a foul odour and of course may contain blood
- Common in females, unusual in males (due to sizes of their respective urethras)
- Catheterisation is a major risk factor as it provides a conduit for bacteria
- In the elderly, the only symptom may be delirium

GLOMERULONEPHRITIS

- Can cause nephritis with frank haematuria, or nephrotic syndrome
- Many different causes; there may be an associated preceding URTI (post-streptococcal or IgA nephropathy); haemoptysis (Goodpasture's syndrome); or systemic features, such as a rash, suggestive of vasculitis

OTHER

- Urinary tract injury – Blunt, penetrating or iatrogenic (e.g. catheterisation)
- Coagulopathy e.g. haemophilia
- Prostatitis
- BPH and prostatic carcinoma (although haematuria not typically seen)
- Beetroot – Turns urine

INVESTIGATIONS

- Urinalysis; culture, microscopy and sensitivity to look for UTIs
- U&Es, FBC and clotting
- eGFR
- Autoantibody screen – ANCA, ANA and anti-glomerular basement membrane
- Urine cytology and cystoscopy for bladder cancer
- USS renal tract to look for masses
- CT kidneys, ureters and bladder if history suggests renal/ureteric colic
- Renal biopsy to confirm glomerulonephritis

MANAGEMENT

- Frank haematuria requires urgent referral on to urology or nephrology
- Bladder cancer – Transurethral resection for superficial tumours; radical cystectomy and urinary diversion for invasive disease; possibly chemotherapy
- Renal cell carcinoma – Nephrectomy
- Renal calculi – <5 mm usually pass on its own; extracorporeal lithotripsy or endoscopic stone removal for medium-sized stones; rarely, intracorporal or open operations are required for larger/persistent stones
- UTI – Antibiotics e.g. trimethoprim in simple uncomplicated cystitis

- Nephrotic syndrome – Treat cause; furosemide, ACE inhibitors and calcium channel blockers to control fluid retention and hypertension
- Rapidly progressive glomerulonephritis requires prompt treatment with high doses of steroids and cyclophosphamide

FURTHER READING

NICE CKS on recognition of urological cancers, http://cks.nice.org.uk/urological-cancers-recognition-and-referral

DYSURIA

INITIATING THE SESSION

- Greet the patient, ask an open question and screen for other problems

MEDICAL PERSPECTIVE

SEQUENCE OF EVENTS

- **Open question** – Can you tell me more about this pain/discomfort?
- **Timeline** – How did it start? How has it progressed since then? Over what period of time has this occurred?

SYMPTOM ANALYSIS (SOCRATES)

- **Site** – Where exactly does it hurt when you pass urine? Is it deep inside or on your skin or genitals?
- **Onset** – When did you first notice the pain?
- **Character** – How would you describe the pain? *Burning*? *Sharp*?
- **Radiation** – Do you get any pain in your abdomen, loin or back? *If so*, does the pain go anywhere else?
- **Associated features** – *See systems review*
- **Timing** – Is the pain there at the start, towards the end or after passing urine? Have you had this pain before?
- **Exacerbating/relieving factors** – Does anything make it better or worse?
- **Severity** – How bad is the pain on a scale of 1–10, with 10 being the worst pain you can imagine?

SYSTEMS REVIEW

RED FLAGS
Haematuria
Weight loss
Rigors
Systemically unwell

- **Frequency** – Are you going to the toilet more frequently? Do you pass large or small volumes of urine?
- **Urgency** – Do you get sudden irrepressible urges to urinate?
- **Haematuria** – Has your urine changed colour? Has there been any blood?
- **Discharge** – Have you noticed any discharge from your vagina/penis? *If so, take full sexual history (see vaginal discharge history, pp. 161)*
- **Constitutional** – Have you been feeling unwell with a fever or shivering? Have you lost any weight?

FOR MALES

- **Prostatism** – Do you have difficulty getting the stream started? Is there prolonged dribbling at the end? Is your stream powerful or weak?
- **Nocturia** – How often do you get up at night to pass urine?
- **Prostatitis** – Do you find ejaculation painful?

FOR FEMALES

- **Menopause** – Have you gone through the change yet? *NB: ask if age appropriate*
- **Dysmenorrhoea** – Is the pain worse during your periods? Does it stop after you have a period?

PATIENT'S PERSPECTIVE

- **Feelings and effect on life** – Have your symptoms had any effect on your daily life?
- **Ideas** – What do you think is causing the pain/discomfort?
- **Concerns** – Is there anything in particular you are concerned could be causing it? Is there anything in general that is concerning you?
- **Expectations** – Was there anything in particular you were hoping for when you made the appointment for today?

BACKGROUND INFORMATION

PMH

- Do you suffer from any medical conditions?
- *Ask about previous UTIs, STIs, renal calculi, catheters and renal tract injury*

DH

- Do you take any medications? Do you have any allergies?

FH

- Do any conditions run in the family? *Ask about any renal/urinary tract problems*

SH

- Do you smoke? Do you drink alcohol? How much?
- Are you working presently? *If so,* what is your job? What does that involve?
- Can you tell me about your home situation (*occupants and any difficulties*)?
- Has your problem affected your job or home life in any way?
- Does your partner have any similar symptoms?

CLOSING THE SESSION

- summary ± examination/explanation and planning/contract

IMPORTANT POINTS

- It is important to tailor this history to the individual e.g. in a 20-year-old female it may not be important to ask about menopause, but taking a sexual history could elucidate key symptoms
- Pain at the start of urination suggests urethritis, but post-voiding, suprapubic pain is suggestive of cystitis

DIFFERENTIAL DIAGNOSIS

URINARY TRACT INFECTION (MOST COMMON)

- Cystitis typically produces urinary frequency, urgency and dysuria
- Fever and suprapubic pain may also be present
- The urine may be cloudy with a foul odour and may contain blood
- More common in women; in the elderly, the only symptom may be delirium

PYELONEPHRITIS (MOST SERIOUS)

- Very unwell – Fever, rigors, nausea, vomiting, flank pain radiating to the back
- Dysuria, frequency, urgency, nocturia and haematuria may be present

SEXUALLY TRANSMITTED INFECTION

- Vaginal/urethral discharge, commonly in young sexually active patients
- Possible history of recent exposure, such as a new partner or unprotected sex
- Possible history of dyspareunia, painful ejaculation or dyschezia (prostatitis)
- Reiter's syndrome (reactive arthritis) – Urethritis, conjunctivitis and arthritis secondary to STI or gastroenteritis; typically, an oligoarthritis

RENAL CALCULI

- Classical presentation – Acute onset of excruciating flank/abdominal pain, radiating from "loin to groin," with associated nausea and vomiting
- Pain in renal colic is more constant than in biliary/intestinal colic, but often periods of relief in which the patient has a dull ache
- Most often however asymptomatic and found incidentally
- Dysuria may be present due to urinary tract damage
- Typically affects men aged between 30 and 50 years

ENDOMETRIOSIS

- Cyclical pelvic pain that peaks before menstruation and then dissipates
- Dyspareunia (deep), dysmenorrhoea, dyschezia, dysuria, subfertility and lower abdominal pain

ATROPHIC VAGINITIS

- Amenorrhoea, poor tissue elasticity and vaginal dryness and pain
- Common in women after menopause and can cause dysuria

BENIGN PROSTATIC HYPERPLASIA

- Urinary frequency and nocturia with obstructive symptoms of hesitancy, terminal dribbling and a weak stream
- Incomplete bladder emptying causes continuous urge to go
- Haematuria may occur; dysuria occurs due to UTI, secondary to urinary stasis

INVESTIGATIONS

- Abdominal examination
- PR examination for older men; consider pelvic examination in women
- Urine analysis
- MSU – culture and sensitivity for UTIs/pyelonephritis
- Bloods – FBC, U&Es, CRP and PSA (older men)
- Blood cultures where pyelonephritis is suspected
- Urethral/high vaginal and endocervical swabs and urine PCR for STIs
- Abdominal USS to detect masses
- CT KUB if suspecting calculi

MANAGEMENT

- UTI – Oral antibiotics as per local guidance in simple uncomplicated cystitis
- Pyelonephritis – Antibiotics e.g. ciprofloxacin; consider admission
- STIs – Refer to genito-urinary medicine; chlamydia and gonorrhoea are best treated with a one-off dose of 1 g azithromycin IM and 500 mg ceftriaxone, respectively; contact tracing should be implemented
- Renal calculi – <5 mm usually pass on its own; extracorporeal lithotripsy or endoscopic stone removal for medium-sized stones; rarely, intracorporal or open operations are required for larger/persistent stones
- BPH – Alpha blockers (e.g. tamsulosin) and 5-alpha reductase inhibitors (e.g. finasteride); transurethral resection of the prostate if medical treatment fails
- Atrophic vaginitis – Topical lubricants; topical oestrogens or pessaries

FURTHER READING

NICE CKS on UTIs, http://cks.nice.org.uk/urinary-tract-infection-lower-women

POLYURIA

INITIATING THE SESSION

- Greet the patient, ask an open question and screen for other problems

MEDICAL PERSPECTIVE

SEQUENCE OF EVENTS

- **Open question** – Can you tell me more about your symptoms?
- **Timeline** – How did it start? How has it progressed since then? Over what period of time has this occurred?

SYMPTOM ANALYSIS

- **Onset** – When did you start to notice this?
- **Frequency** – How many times do you pass urine a day? More than six times?
- **Nocturia** – How often do you get up at night to pass urine? More than twice?
- **Amount** – How much do you pass each time? Is it large or small amounts?
- **Thirst** – Are you thirsty? How much fluid do you drink in a day?

SYSTEMS REVIEW

- **Dysuria** – Does it hurt or burn to pass urine?
- **Haematuria/discharge** – Have you noticed any change in the colour of your urine? Is there any blood or discharge? *If so,* can you describe it please?
- **Urge incontinence** – Do you ever get a sudden irrepressible urge to pass water? Are you able to hold it in when this happens?
- **Abdo pain** – Have you had any pain in your abdomen?
- **Constitutional** – Have you felt feverish? Have you had chills and shivers with it (*rigors*)? Have you had any recent weight loss? How is your appetite?

FOR MALES

- **Prostatism** – Do you have difficulty getting your stream started? Is there prolonged dribbling at the end? Is your stream powerful or weak?

FOR FEMALES

- **Prolapse** – Do you have a feeling of fullness or a dropping sensation from your pelvis? Does anything protrude from your vagina e.g. when you open your bowels or strain?
- **Obstetric history** – How many children have you had? How were they born (vaginal vs. caesarean)? Were they large babies?
- **Menopause** – Have you gone through the change yet?

PATIENT'S PERSPECTIVE

- **Feelings and effect on life** – Have your symptoms had any effect on your daily life?
- **Ideas** – What do you think is causing you to pass urine more frequently?
- **Concerns** – Is there anything in particular you are concerned could be causing it? Is there anything in general that is concerning you?
- **Expectations** – Was there anything in particular you were hoping for when you made the appointment for today?

BACKGROUND INFORMATION

PMH

- Do you suffer from any medical conditions?
- *Ask specifically about diabetes*

DH

- Do you take any regular medication? Do you have any allergies?
- *Ask specifically about diuretics*

FH

- Do any conditions run in your family?
- *Ask specifically about diabetes and renal conditions generally*

SH

- Do you smoke? Drink alcohol? How much?
- Are you currently working? *If so,* what is your job? What does that involve?
- Can you tell me about your home situation (*occupants and any difficulties*)?
- Has your problem affected your job or home life in any way?

CLOSING THE SESSION

- summary ± examination/explanation and planning/contract

IMPORTANT POINTS

- Polyuria is defined objectively as the production of more than 3 litres of urine in 24 hours, although in practice finding out the exact volume of urine they are passing from the history is often not possible – It may be necessary to get a voiding diary detailing frequency and volumes of urination
- Again, tailor the history to the patient sitting in front of you – In a young woman the gynaecological history may not be as important as it is in elderly patients, and it may not be appropriate to ask about menopause in such patients

DIFFERENTIAL DIAGNOSIS

URINARY TRACT INFECTION (MOST COMMON)

- Cystitis typically produces urinary frequency, urgency and dysuria
- Fever, suprapubic pain and urethral discharge may also be present
- The urine may be cloudy with a foul odour and may contain blood
- More common in women; in the elderly, the only symptom may be delirium

DIABETES MELLITUS (MOST SERIOUS)

- Polydipsia and polyuria, with abdominal pain, nausea, vomiting, weight loss and "pear drop" breath seen in diabetic ketoacidosis
- May be presenting feature, particularly in type 1 diabetes mellitus
- Often a family history of diabetes

HYPERACTIVE BLADDER

- Severe urgency, nocturia, frequency and possibly incontinence
- There may be a past history of neurological conditions such as Parkinson's disease, stroke or spinal cord disease

GENITO-URINARY PROLAPSE

- Common among older women
- Risk factors include multiple vaginal deliveries, menopause, obesity, complicated vaginal deliveries and hysterectomy
- Symptoms include urinary frequency, recurrent UTIs, stress or urge incontinence and a fullness sensation in the vagina

BENIGN PROSTATIC HYPERPLASIA

- Urinary frequency and nocturia with obstructive symptoms of hesitancy, terminal dribbling and a weak stream
- Incomplete bladder emptying causes continuous urge to pass urine
- Haematuria and dysuria may also occur

DIABETES INSIPIDUS

- Polydipsia and polyuria
- Patients produce huge quantities of very dilute urine (almost pure water); they are rarely dehydrated unless prevented from drinking large quantities of water
- Nocturia is often present and bothersome; however, there are no symptoms suggestive of an obstructive or irritative urinary disorder
- Can be inherited, presenting within the first few years of life

OTHERS

- Iatrogenic – Diuretics used to treat hypertension are a very common cause
- Psychogenic polydipsia – Patient drinks beyond true water requirement; more common nowadays due to the belief that drinking lots of water is healthy

- Hypercalcaemia – Abdominal pain, vomiting, drowsiness, confusion, anorexia, muscle weakness and constipation; malignancy, Paget's disease of bone and hyperparathyroidism or all recognised causes
- Hypokalaemia – Non-specific symptoms of constipation, weakness and confusion; augmented by diarrhoea, vomiting, diuretics and laxative abuse

INVESTIGATIONS

- Abdominal examination
- PR examination for older men; consider pelvic examination in women
- FBC, U&Es, fasting glucose and PSA (older men)
- Urine osmolality to see if it is a solute or water diuresis
- Urine analysis
- MSU sample – culture and sensitivity
- Urodynamic investigation
- Water deprivation test

MANAGEMENT

- UTI – Oral antibiotics as per local guidance in simple uncomplicated cystitis
- Diabetes mellitus – Insulin regime for type 1 diabetics; diet-controlled or treated with metformin (and possibly hypoglycaemics) for type 2 diabetics
- In diabetic ketoacidosis, emergency admission with fluid and electrolyte resuscitation is required initially, with insulin until glucose level is controlled
- Diabetes insipidus – Careful regular fluid intake may suffice in mild cases; exogenous antidiuretic hormone is given where this is not sufficient
- Genito-urinary prolapse – Vaginal pessaries; surgery to tighten and reattach the pelvic ligaments in younger patients or where pessaries aren't sufficient
- BPH – Alpha blockers (e.g. tamsulosin) and 5-alpha reductase inhibitors (e.g. finasteride); transurethral resection of the prostate if medical treatment fails
- Hyperactive bladder – Pelvic floor exercises; cutting out caffeine and alcohol; anticholinergics (e.g. oxybutynin); surgery e.g. sacral nerve stimulation or intravesical botulinum toxin may be considered in refractory cases
- Diuretics (iatrogenic) – Take once in the morning to avoid disturbed nights
- Hypercalcaemia – Treat cause; fluids; bisphosphonates; loop diuretics
- Hypokalaemia – Treat cause; the severity of the deficit and clinical findings dictate whether intensive replacement or conservative measures are necessary

FURTHER READING

NICE CKS on lower urinary tract symptoms in men, http://cks.nice.org.uk/luts-in-men

Ear, nose and throat

DIZZINESS AND VERTIGO

INITIATING THE SESSION

- Greet the patient, ask an open question and screen for other problems

MEDICAL PERSPECTIVE

SEQUENCE OF EVENTS AND SYMPTOM ANALYSIS

- **Open question** – Can you tell me more about your dizziness?
- **Specify** – What exactly do you mean when you say you feel "dizzy"?
- **Timeline** – Tell me about the first time it happened. What were you doing at the time? How long did it last for? Have all the attacks been the same since? Is it there all the time or does it come and go? Does it come on suddenly or slowly?
- **Triggers** – Does anything bring it on? Is it brought on by turning your head in one direction or the other? Does it happen when lying down in bed? Does it happen when you try to stand up? *If so*, do you ever get it when you are sitting down? Does anything make it better or worse?

SYSTEMS REVIEW

- **Hearing** – Have you noticed any change in your hearing?
- **Ears** – Have you had any earache? Any discharge? Any ringing in your ears?
- **Sensory** – Do you have any numbness/tingling anywhere? Have you noticed any changes in vision or eye pain?
- **Motor** – Any feelings of weakness? Any difficulty with daily activities?
- **Speech** – Have you had any trouble with your speech previously?
- **Headaches** – Have you suffered from any bad headaches or migraines recently?
- **Falls and blackouts** – Has it caused you to fall or have any blackouts?
- **Constitutional** – Have you noticed any weight loss? Any fever? Any nausea or vomiting?

> **RED FLAGS**
>
> *Prolonged/severe vertigo*
> *Headache*
> *Neurological symptoms*

PATIENT'S PERSPECTIVE

- **Feelings and effect on life** – How has your dizziness affected your day-to-day life?
- **Ideas** – Do you have any ideas yourself about what could be the cause of the dizziness?
- **Concerns** – Is there anything you are particularly concerned could be causing the dizziness? Is there anything in general that concerns you?
- **Expectations** – Was there anything in particular you were hoping for when you made the appointment today, other than trying to get to the bottom of it?

BACKGROUND INFORMATION

PMH

- Do you suffer from any medical conditions?
- *Ask specifically about previous strokes, recent infections and recent trauma*

DH

- Are you taking any medications? Have any of these been changed recently?
- Do you have any allergies?

FH

- Do any conditions run in the family?

SH

- Do you drink alcohol? *If so,* how much? Are you under the influence of alcohol when the dizziness comes on?
- Do you smoke? How many cigarettes do you smoke a day? For how long?
- Do you take any recreational drugs?
- Are you currently working? *If so,* what is your job? What does that involve?
- Can you tell me about your home situation (*occupants and any difficulties*)?
- Has your problem affected your job or home life?

CLOSING THE SESSION

- summary ± examination/explanation and planning/contract

IMPORTANT POINTS

- "Dizziness" can mean different things to different people – It is important to clarify early on exactly what the patient means by the term. Does the patient feel as if the room is spinning around them? Do they feel like they are going to faint? Do they simply feel unsteady on their feet and fall over? (*see falls history pp. 6*)
- Vertigo is the sensation that the patient or the room they are in is spinning, often coupled with nausea and nystagmus
- In pre-syncope the patient may be feeling faint or light-headed
- Feelings of dizziness can also be of psychiatric origin

DIFFERENTIAL DIAGNOSIS

Whilst arriving at a correct diagnosis can often be challenging initially, it is important to decipher whether the cause of the vertigo is a central one (i.e. central nervous system) or peripheral (inner ear). Central vertigo tends to last longer, is more intense and is usually associated with other neurological symptoms. Peripheral vertigo tends to improve with time, whereas central causes tend not to.

PERIPHERAL VERTIGO

BENIGN PAROXYSMAL POSITIONAL VERTIGO

- Usually only lasts for seconds and is precipitated by looking up and to one side – classically occurs when lying down in bed
- No deafness or tinnitus
- Usually asymptomatic between attacks

ACUTE LABYRINTHITIS/VESTIBULAR NEURONITIS

- Sudden onset
- Acute attack lasts for days – typically patients have 3 days of acute attack, 3 weeks of being unsteady and 3 months before they are back to normal. This is the timescale for the initial insult and then for compensation to take place.
- Can be severe with difficulty staying on their feet as well as nausea and vomiting
- In acute labyrinthitis there is deafness, whereas in vestibular neuronitis there is no deafness
- Can be viral or vascular in origin

MENIERE'S DISEASE

- Triad of vertigo, tinnitus and progressive hearing loss (usually unilateral)
- Usually preceded by a warning i.e. feeling of fullness in the ear
- Attacks usually last up to a few hours
- Weakly associated with high-salt diets and alcohol, caffeine and tobacco consumption

OTOTOXICITY

- Streptomycin, vancomycin, gentamycin, chloroquines and chemotherapy are all potentially ototoxic drugs
- Deafness and tinnitus

HERPES ZOSTER OTICUS (RAMSAY HUNT SYNDROME)

- Shingles; reactivation of varicella zoster in the geniculate ganglion of the facial nerve
- They commonly present with an extremely painful and blistered external meatus
- Facial palsy, deafness and tinnitus may also present

CENTRAL VERTIGO (*See Red Flags*)

STROKE/ TRANSIENT ISCHAEMIC ATTACK

- Other neurological symptoms present
- Elderly with other risk factors for stroke
- Severe, persistent symptoms with severe imbalance

VESTIBULAR MIGRAINE

- Lasts from minutes to hours or even days
- Increasingly recognised as a cause for episodic vertigo
- Can mimic Meniere's disease but without progressive hearing loss
- Usually past history of classical migraine
- Usually cannot tolerate being a passenger in a car
- Eased by sleep and rest and brought on with stress

OTHER

- Multiple sclerosis
- Head injury
- Intracranial haemorrhage

INVESTIGATIONS

- Full otoneurological examination, including cranial nerves and gait assessment
- Eye examination for nystagmus
- Otoscopy
- Dix–Hallpike test for BPPV
- Audiometry
- ECG
- CT/MRI head if neurology found or concern regarding central cause of vertigo

MANAGEMENT

- General – Review medication and stop ototoxic drugs; consider risk towards driving and occupational hazards; treat vertigo and nausea acutely with anti-emetics (e.g. prochlorperazine – this should only be prescribed for short courses)
- BPPV – Epley manoeuvre
- Acute labyrinthitis – Bed rest and anti-emetics initially then gradually build up daily routine with assistance once managing to get out of bed
- Meniere's disease – Diet low in salt and avoiding alcohol, caffeine and tobacco may help prevent attacks; prophylactic betahistine and diuretics may be of benefit; anti-emetics for acute attacks; hearing aid(s) if required; surgery if these options fail
- Herpes zoster oticus – Analgesia, aciclovir and prednisolone

FURTHER READING

NICE CKS on vertigo, http://cks.nice.org.uk/vertigo

NECK LUMPS

INITIATING THE SESSION

- Greet the patient, ask an open question and screen for other problems

MEDICAL PERSPECTIVE

SEQUENCE OF EVENTS AND SYMPTOM ANALYSIS

- **Open question** – Can you tell me more about this lump?
- **Site** – Where exactly is the lump? Can you point to it?
- **Timeline** – When did you first notice the lump? Has it changed over time? Is it getting bigger or smaller?
- **Tenderness** – Is it painful to touch?
- **Other lumps** – Are there any other similar lumps that you have noticed?
- **Previous episodes** – Have you ever had a similar lump before? *If so,* what happened?

SYSTEMS REVIEW

- **ENT** – Have you had any difficulty swallowing? Is it painful to swallow? Does thinking about or tasting food cause pain? Have you noticed a hoarse voice? Have you had any earache? Have you noticed a sore throat or a cold recently?
- **RS** – Do you have a cough? *If so,* do you bring anything up? Any blood? Have you found yourself more breathless than previously?
- **Haematological** – Have you been more prone to bruising or bleeding recently? Have you been having recurrent infections? Have you noticed any pain in your bones?
- **Constitutional** – Have you noticed any weight loss? Have you felt overly tired? Have you felt feverish? Have you had drenching night sweats? Have you travelled abroad in the last 6 months?
- **Trauma** – Have you had any trauma to the area?

> **RED FLAGS**
>
> *Weight loss*
> *Night sweats*
> *Heavy smoking history*
> *Dysphagia*
> *Odynophagia*
> *Hoarseness >3 weeks*
> *Unexplained bruising*
> *Recurrent infections*

PATIENT'S PERSPECTIVE

- **Feelings and effect on life** – Finding a lump can be a frightening experience. How has this affected you?
- **Ideas** – Do you have any ideas yourself about what could be causing your symptoms?
- **Concerns** – Is there anything you are particularly concerned could be causing it? Is there anything in general that concerns you?
- **Expectations** – Would I be right in thinking that you have come in today mainly to try to find out what is causing it? Was there anything else you were hoping for today?

BACKGROUND INFORMATION

PMH

- Do you suffer from any medical conditions? *Ask specifically about past lymphoma*

DH

- Are you taking any medications? Do you have any allergies?

FH

- Has anyone else in your family suffered from similar problems?

SH

- Do you smoke? How many cigarettes do you smoke a day? For how long?
- Do you drink alcohol? How much do you drink in a week?
- Are you currently working? *If so,* what is your job? What does that involve?
- Can you tell me about your home situation (*occupants and any difficulties*)?
- Has your problem affected your job or home life in any way?
- Has anyone at home or at work been ill with anything recently? *If so, specify*

CLOSING THE SESSION

- summary ± examination/explanation and planning/contract

> **IMPORTANT POINTS**
>
> - This is likely to be a combined history and examination station, in which most of the time will be spent on the examination aspect. If given sufficient time for a history, you may wish to enquire about every aspect of the history, but in most cases it will suffice to focus on the medical perspective
> - Always consider whether the lump could represent a malignancy and ask relevant questions to help determine the likelihood of this (e.g. weight loss, non-tender lump, previous cancer, heavy smoking history etc.)

DIFFERENTIAL DIAGNOSIS

Lymphadenopathy refers to nodes that are abnormal in size, consistency or number and can be either "localised" or "generalised" if more than one group is affected. Lymph nodes are generally considered normal up to 1 cm in diameter, apart from the jugulodigastric node, which can be up to 1.5 cm.

REACTIVE LYMPHADENOPATHY (MOST COMMON)

- May last up to 4 weeks and are usually associated with signs and symptoms of a local infection relative to the affected lymph node e.g. tonsillitis to level 2 (jugulodigastric) lymph nodes
- Reactive lymph nodes tend to be regular, soft-to-firm on palpation and mobile

METASTATIC CARCINOMA (MOST SERIOUS)

- Head and neck malignancies metastasise to cervical nodes relative to their location
- Persistent hoarseness, sore throat, pain on swallowing, cough or sensation of lump in the throat could suggest an underlying head and neck tumour

- Smoking, alcohol and old age are risk factors for head and neck malignancies
- Cancerous nodes are typically hard and irregular when palpated

LYMPHOMA

- B symptoms of weight loss, drenching night sweats and fever may be present
- The lymph nodes are typically firm and rubbery to palpate
- Hodgkin's lymphoma, more common in adulthood, has two peaks of incidence – age 20–25 years and >70 years, but can occur at any age

TUBERCULOSIS

- Affected lymph nodes may be large
- Long-standing fever, malaise, weight loss and night sweats (classically)
- A history of foreign travel or contact with someone who has TB may well be given
- Other risk factors include immunosuppression, alcoholism and IV drug users

SIALOLITHIASIS (SALIVARY GLAND OBSTRUCTION)

- Intermittent and post-prandial pain and swelling in the submandibular or parotid gland
- May be provoked by dehydration
- Can get secondary infection with redness, pain and potentially abscess formation

BRANCHIAL CYST

- Congenital epithelial cyst that arises on the lateral part of the neck
- Smooth, soft and non-tender; usually presents in the second or third decade of life as a smooth, slowly enlarging lateral neck mass that may increase in size after an upper respiratory tract infection

CYSTIC HYGROMA

- Congenital multiloculated lymphatic lesion that presents either on antenatal scanning, at birth or in the first 2 years of life
- Classically found in the left posterior triangle of the neck

EPIDERMOID CYST (AKA SEBACEOUS CYST)

- Sebaceous cysts are intradermal (skin cannot be drawn over them)
- They have a characteristic punctum
- They most commonly appear on the face, trunk, neck, extremities and the scalp
- Commonly become infected, causing a tender lump with discharge from the punctum

ABSCESS

- Red, hot and fluctuant swelling in a feverish patient
- Local spread

THYROID SWELLING/GOITRE

- Hypothyroidism and hyperthyroidism can cause different types of goitre, although most people with a goitre are euthyroid
- Moves on swallowing
- Thyroglossal duct cysts move with protrusion of the tongue

PAROTITIS

- Can be due to infection (bacterial or mumps), autoimmune problems (e.g. Sjogren's syndrome) or obstruction (e.g. sialolithiasis)
- Swelling of parotid gland causing pain and enlargement of the gland

CAROTID ARTERY ANEURYSM

- Large, pulsatile mass when palpating carotid artery; rare

CAROTID BODY TUMOUR

- Occurs at bifurcation of carotids
- Can be associated with other tumours

INVESTIGATIONS

- Clinical examination of all lymph nodes in neck, axilla and groin
- Bloods including FBC and blood film for unexplained lymphadenopathy
- If lymph node is concerning for malignancy, urgent referral to ENT required
- If highly likely to be benign, watchful monitoring is appropriate for 1 month
- CXR for supraclavicular lymphadenopathy
- Imaging via ultrasound scan, CT or MRI
- Fine needle aspiration
- Core or excision biopsy

MANAGEMENT

- A 4-week observation period is appropriate if likely benign lymphadenopathy
- Head and neck cancer – Urgent referral; surgery, chemotherapy and/or radiotherapy
- Lymphoma – Chemotherapy
- Tuberculosis – 6 months treatment with isoniazid and rifampicin with the addition for the first 2 months of pyrazinamide and ethambutol
- Sialolithiasis – Hydration, massage, citrus, basket retrieval, shock wave therapy, surgery
- Goitre – Dependent on cause and symptoms as may be asymptomatic; thyroxine replacement, radioactive iodine, surgery
- Sebaceous cyst, branchial cyst and cystic hygroma – Excision if problematic
- Abscess – Incision and adequate drainage
- Parotitis – Antibiotics if infective in nature

FURTHER READING

NICE CKS on neck lumps, http://cks.nice.org.uk/neck-lump

EARACHE

INITIATING THE SESSION

- Greet the patient, ask an open question and screen for other problems

MEDICAL PERSPECTIVE

SEQUENCE OF EVENTS AND SYMPTOM ANALYSIS (SOCRATES)

- **Open question** – Can you tell me more about your earache?
- **Site** – Which ear have you noticed the problem in? How is the other ear?
- **Onset** – When did you first notice this? How have the symptoms changed over time?
- **Character** – What does the pain feel like?
- **Radiation** – Does the pain go anywhere else? Do you have a sore throat?
- **Associated features** – *See systems review*
- **Timing** – Is the pain always there or does it come and go?
- **Exacerbating/relieving factors** – Does anything make it better or worse?
- **Severity** – How bad is the pain on a scale of 1 to 10?

SYSTEMS REVIEW

RED FLAGS

Diabetes
Old age
Neurological symptoms
Persistent
Weight loss

- **Otorrhoea** – Have you had any discharge from either ear? *If so,* what colour/consistency is it?
- **Itch** – Do your ears feel itchy?
- **Vertigo** – Have you had episodes where it feels as if the room is spinning around you? Any difficulties with your balance?
- **Tinnitus** – Have you noticed a ringing in your ears?
- **Foreign bodies** – Do you ever clean your ears with cotton buds or anything else?
- **NS** – Do you have a headache? Any neck stiffness? Rash? Photophobia? Any numbness or tingling anywhere? Any new muscle weakness?
- **Constitutional** – Have you felt ill or feverish recently? Any weight loss?

PATIENT'S PERSPECTIVE

- **Feelings and effect on life** – How have your symptoms affected your life?
- **Ideas** – Do you have any ideas yourself about what could be causing your earache?
- **Concerns** – Is there anything you are particularly concerned could be causing it? Is there anything in general that concerns you?
- **Expectations** – Was there anything in particular you were hoping for when you made the appointment to come see me today?

BACKGROUND INFORMATION

PMH

- Do you suffer from any medical conditions? Have you had any surgery on your ears before?

DH

- Are you currently taking any medications? Have you tried any medications to help so far? Do you have any allergies?

FH

- Do any conditions run in your family?

SH

- Do you smoke? How many cigarettes do you smoke a day? For how long?
- Do you drink alcohol? How much do you drink in a week?
- Are you currently working? *If so,* what is your job? What does that involve?
- Can you tell me about your home situation (*occupants and any difficulties)?*
- Has your problem affected your job or home life in any way?

CLOSING THE SESSION

- summary ± examination/explanation and planning/contract

> **IMPORTANT POINTS**
>
> - It is important to ascertain whether the symptoms are unilateral or bilateral, recurrent and what treatment has already been tried
> - The vast majority of these cases present in general practice and are benign in nature, but it is important to screen for the serious pathology by asking about neurological symptoms
> - Children with seizures in the presence of an otitis media should *not* be given a diagnosis of febrile convulsions without ENT specialist assessment + imaging

DIFFERENTIAL DIAGNOSIS

OTITIS EXTERNA

- Itchy, painful ear with discharge
- Itch comes on first followed by watery discharge then pain and finally hearing loss
- Often a history of recurrent similar infections, use of cotton buds and skin conditions such as eczema
- Beware of the elderly diabetic patients with pain out of proportion to clinical findings – they may have necrotising otitis externa, where the infection spreads to the base of skull; they need an acute referral to ENT if this is suspected

ACUTE OTITIS MEDIA

- Common in children <10 y/o in particular
- Hearing loss and severe pain comes first followed by thick purulent discharge and a resolution of pain as ear drum bursts

- Classic history of toddler initially with URTI, then high temp, screaming through the night, then blood-stained foul ear discharge and a peaceful child that is no longer in any distress. Toddlers/infants may simply present with irritability and/or pulling at their ear
- Unable to "pop" ears and will have decreased hearing in that ear
- Commonly self-limiting but can lead to severe complications rarely such as mastoiditis and meningitis

OTITIS MEDIA WITH EFFUSION (GLUE EAR)

- Longer history
- Hearing difficulty tends to be the predominant feature
- Pain is usually milder if present at all

CHRONIC SUPPURATIVE OTITIS MEDIA

- Chronic inflammation of the middle ear, presenting with recurrent discharge through a perforated tympanic membrane
- Otorrhoea present >2 weeks without pain or fever

EAR WAX

- The vast majority of earwax will cause no problem at all even if extensive
- Decreased hearing ± mild pain only occurs if patients have been manipulating the EAC/wax or wax has been syringed and a subsequent otitis externa has taken hold
- The patient may admit to use of cotton buds

REFERRED PAIN FROM OROPHARYNX

- Patients can get referred pain in either ear from the pharynx e.g. tonsillitis
- If it doesn't resolve and no cause is found, specialist ENT input is needed

INVESTIGATIONS

- No investigations are usually required for simple otitis media/externa
- In cases of treatment failure in otitis externa, an ear swab can be taken
- Audiometry and tympanometry may be required in glue ear
- CT/MRI if neurological symptoms or concern about necrotising otitis externa, mastoiditis or meningeal spread

MANAGEMENT

- Otitis externa – topical antibiotics with steroid; if the canal is very oedematous or there is significant debris it may be necessary to refer to ENT for aural cleaning and/or pope wick placement
- Acute otitis media – oral antibiotics if not resolved after 4 days or meets other criteria according to NICE guidelines (can be issued as a delayed script)
- Glue ear – Grommets or hearing aids if not resolving and conductive hearing loss on audiometry

- Chronic suppurative otitis media – Refer to ENT for management, which may include aural cleaning, topical antibiotic therapy and/or surgery
- Hearing aids if hearing does not improve after other measures
- Ear wax – Olive oil ear drops ± ear syringing or microsuction of wax
- Necrotising otitis externa – IV antibiotics with aural cleaning
- Mastoiditis/meningitis – IV antibiotics ± surgical management later

FURTHER READING

NICE CKS on:

Otitis externa, http://cks.nice.org.uk/otitis-externa

Acute otitis media, http://cks.nice.org.uk/otitis-media-acute

Otitis media with effusion, http://cks.nice.org.uk/otitis-media-with-effusion

Chronic suppurative otitis media, http://cks.nice.org.uk/otitis-media-chronic-suppurative

HEARING IMPAIRMENT (ADULT)

INITIATING THE SESSION

- Greet the patient, ask an open question and screen for other problems

MEDICAL PERSPECTIVE

SEQUENCE OF EVENTS AND SYMPTOM ANALYSIS

- **Open question** – What exactly have you noticed?
- **Side** – Is one ear better than the other or are both affected? Which ear did it start in?
- **Timeline** – When did you first notice this? Has it changed over time? Did it come on suddenly or gradually? *If suddenly,* what were you doing at the time? *(Barotrauma – E.g. deep sea diving, sudden explosive noises and head trauma)*
- **Environment** – Do you find any particular noises hard to hear? Do you have difficulty hearing in background noise?

SYSTEMS REVIEW

- **Vertigo** – Do you ever feel as if the room is spinning around you?
- **Otorrhoea** – Do you get any discharge from your ears?
- **Tinnitus** – Do you get a ringing noise in either ear?
- **Foreign bodies** – Do you ever clean your ears with cotton buds or anything else?
- **Balance** – Any problems with your balance?
- **Sensory** – Any numbness or tingling anywhere (particularly in the face)?
- **Motor** – Any feelings of weakness (particularly in the face)?
- **Headaches** – Do you have a headache?
- **Infection** – Have you felt ill or feverish recently? *Postinfective hearing loss – herpes, influenza, syphilis, measles, mumps, meningitis, rubella, CMV*
- **Constitutional** – Have you noticed any weight loss? How has your appetite been? Have you been feeling tired?

RED FLAGS

Neurological symptoms
Trauma
Sudden onset
Severity
Weight loss

PATIENT'S PERSPECTIVE

- **Feelings and effect on life** – How has your hearing loss affected you?
- **Ideas** – Do you have any ideas yourself about what could be causing it?
- **Concerns** – Is there anything you are particularly concerned could be causing it? Is there anything in general that concerns you?
- **Expectations** – Other than trying to get to the bottom of why it has happened, was there anything in particular you were hoping for when you made the appointment?

BACKGROUND INFORMATION

PMH

- Do you suffer from any medical conditions? Have you had any surgery on your ears?

DH

- Are you taking any medications?
- *Ask specifically about antibiotics (streptomycin, vancomycin and gentamycin) and chemotherapy*
- Do you have any allergies?

FH

- Do any conditions run in your family?
- Any problems with deafness in the family? *If so,* what age did the family member become deaf? Did they have any other problems (tinnitus, vertigo, other neurology)?

SH

- What hobbies do you have? Do you listen to loud music or attend rock concerts?
- Are you currently working? *If so,* what is your job? What does that involve? Did this involve any exposure to loud noises?
- Can you tell me about your home situation (*occupants and any difficulties)?*
- Has your problem affected your job or home life in any way?
- How much alcohol do you drink?
- Do you smoke? How many do/did you smoke? How many years for?

CLOSING THE SESSION

- summary ± examination/explanation and planning/contract

IMPORTANT POINTS

- When speaking to someone who is hard of hearing, it is important to clarify at the beginning of the consultation how easy it will be to communicate
- To aid communication, try to find if one ear is better than the other, decrease background noise and sit at the same level so they can see your mouth moving
- Try to pick short sentences when asking questions, speak loudly and clearly; you may need to arrange for a sign language translator to be present
- The presence or absence of tinnitus, vertigo, balance and other neurological symptoms will aid diagnosis
- The social history can delineate many causes of hearing loss/tinnitus e.g. attending loud rock concerts, working with pneumatic drills etc.

DIFFERENTIAL DIAGNOSIS

CONDUCTIVE HEARING LOSS

External canal pathology (most common)

- Wax or foreign bodies such as the tips of cotton buds
- Infective causes such as otitis externa

Nasopharyngeal tumour (most serious)

- Can cause eustachian tube blockage causing symptoms below:
    - Gradual unilateral hearing loss, repeated infections and a feeling of fullness in the ear
    - Local effects – Headache, mandibular immobility, facial numbness and nosebleeds

Tympanic membrane perforation

- Often due to rapid pressure changes such as on a plane, diving or an explosion; can also be due to infection and trauma
- Perforation needs to be large to cause hearing loss

Otitis media with effusion (glue ear)

- Glue ear is the commonest cause of hearing loss in childhood
- Mild earache may also be present, with fluid accumulation in the middle ear

Otosclerosis

- Hearing loss starting in early adult life; 85% bilateral; female to male ratio 2:1
- 75% also complain of tinnitus
- 50% have family history (autosomal dominant with incomplete penetrance)
- Worsens in menstruation, pregnancy and menopause and improves with background noise

Cholesteatoma

- This is a misnomer; it has nothing to do with cholesterol and is not a tumour
- Non-malignant epithelial growth which often becomes infected
- Can be congenital but most commonly acquired
- Repeated episodes of purulent discharge usually over a number of months or even years with progressive unilateral deafness
- Local effects such as headache, facial nerve palsy, pain and vertigo may also be present and are concerning for intracranial extension/complications

SENSORINEURAL HEARING LOSS

PRESBYCUSIS

- Gradual loss of hearing starting with high-frequency sounds from age 30 years
- Normally occurs in both ears but can be to different extents
- Worse with background noise or when multiple people are speaking
- Not normally a problem until later life when certain high-frequency vocal sounds cannot be heard

MENIERE'S DISEASE

- Progressive deafness
- Attacks of vertigo with nausea, tinnitus and a feeling of ear fullness occur in clusters
- Associated with high-salt diets and alcohol, caffeine and tobacco consumption

OTHER CAUSES OF HEARING LOSS

- Sudden sensorineural loss can be due to numerous causes (surgical sieve) and requires prompt ENT referral and investigation
- Medications
- Post-infectious
- Environmental (noise)
- Multiple sclerosis
- Acoustic neuroma, metastases or another primary brain tumour
- Stroke (rare)
- Vasculitis (rare)

INVESTIGATIONS

- Full neurological and ENT examination with Rinne's and Weber's tests
- Otoscopy
- Audiometry
- Bloods – Gentamycin level (if relevant), FBC, U&Es, LFTs, CRP and ESR
- CT/MRI
- Biopsy of nasopharyngeal lesions and local lymph nodes

MANAGEMENT

- Review medications e.g. gentamycin, and general measures e.g. avoiding loud concerts and any occupational hazards where possible
- If sudden sensorineural hearing loss, start oral steroids and refer to ENT
- Earwax – Ear drops (e.g. olive oil); irrigation or microsuction if available
- Glue ear – Watchful waiting; consider adenoidectomy and grommets e.g. if prolonged history (>3 months)
- Tympanic membrane perforation – Watchful waiting; antibiotics if infected; tympanoplasty if symptomatic and fails to heal by itself
- Otosclerosis – Surgery – stapedectomy or stapedotomy; hearing aids
- Cholesteatoma – Surgery to remove cholesteatoma and topical antibiotics
- Meniere's disease – Patient to inform DVLA; anti-emetics for attacks; prophylaxis – avoid caffeine, alcohol and tobacco; prophylactic betahistine; hearing aids
- Hearing aids depending on audiometry if other methods fail to restore hearing

FURTHER READING

Patient.co.uk professional article on hearing loss, http://patient.info/doctor/deafness-in-adults NICE are producing some guidance on the subject to be released in May 2018.

SORE THROAT

INITIATING THE SESSION

- Greet the patient, ask an open question and screen for other problems

MEDICAL PERSPECTIVE

SEQUENCE OF EVENTS AND SYMPTOM ANALYSIS (SOCRATES)

- **Open question** – Can you tell me more about your sore throat?
- **Site** – Where exactly are you getting the pain? Can you point to it?
- **Onset** – When did you first notice it? How did your symptoms start? How have things changed since it started? Is the sore throat getting any better or worse?
- **Character** – *Less relevant here*
- **Radiation** – Does the pain go anywhere else e.g. to your ears?
- **Asssociated features** – *See systems review*
- **Timing** – Is the sore throat always there?
- **Exacerbating/relieving factors** – Does anything make the pain better or worse?
- **Severity** – Has the pain stopped you from being able to eat or drink?

SYSTEMS REVIEW

- **Constitutional** – Have you felt feverish? Have you felt more tired than you would consider normal? *If older and persistent,* have you lost any weight?
- **Airway** – Have you had any difficulty breathing? Has your voice changed in any way?
- **Neck** – Do you find it difficult moving your neck? Have you noticed any lumps in your neck?
- **URTI** – Have you noticed a cough? Runny nose?

RED FLAGS

Stridor
Drooling
Dyspnoea
Trismus
Neck stiffness
Muffled voice
Persistent sore throat
Smoking, alcohol

PATIENT'S PERSPECTIVE

- **Feelings and effect on life** – How have your symptoms affected you?
- **Ideas** – Do you have any ideas yourself about what could be causing the sore throat?
- **Concerns** – Is there anything you are particularly concerned could be causing it? Is there anything in general that concerns you?
- **Expectations** – Was there anything in particular you were hoping for when you made the appointment for today?

BACKGROUND INFORMATION

PMH

- Do you suffer from any medical conditions?
- Have you had similar problems before? Do you suffer from tonsillitis often? *If so,* how many times have you had it in the past year?

DH

- Are you taking any medications? Do you have any allergies?
- What treatment have you tried so far for it?

FH

- Do any conditions run in your family?

SH

- Do you drink alcohol? How much alcohol do you drink in a week?
- Do you smoke? How many do/did you smoke? How many years for?
- Are you currently working? *If so,* what is your job? What does that involve?
- Can you tell me about your home situation (*occupants and any difficulties)?*
- Has your problem affected your job or home life in any way?

CLOSING THE SESSION

- summary ± examination/explanation and planning/contract

> **IMPORTANT POINTS**
>
> - It is important to ascertain how the sore throat has affected them. If they are able to eat and drink and have no red flags (the vast majority of cases) then you can safely manage the patient in the community.
> - Sore throat is common in younger individuals, but in older individuals you should always consider whether or not there could be an underlying malignancy.

DIFFERENTIAL DIAGNOSIS

PHARYNGITIS (MOST COMMON)

- Common with self-limiting viral URTIs
- May also have a cough, runny/blocked nose, "blocked" ears and headache

SUPRAGLOTTITIS/EPIGLOTTITIS (MOST SERIOUS)

- Sore throat, fever, muffled voice and decreased range of neck movement
- Stridor, drooling and dyspnoea are worrying features
- Epiglottitis is less common since the introduction of the Hib vaccine
- Commonly it is suspected where the symptoms do not fit with the clinical picture (e.g. severe sore throat and odynophagia in the absence of a significant tonsillitis)

TONSILLITIS

- Sore throat may radiate to respective ear
- Previous episodes (if >5 episodes per year refer for tonsillectomy)
- May be viral or bacterial
- CENTOR criteria are useful in determining the likelihood of the sore throat being due to bacterial infection (1 point for each) – Absence of cough; fever; tender anterior cervical lymphadenopathy; and tonsillar exudate. A score of 3 or 4 gives a positive predictive value of roughly 50%

INFECTIOUS MONONUCLEOSIS (GLANDULAR FEVER)

- Mimics tonsillitis
- Viral condition (Epstein–Barr virus) causing sore throat, fever, fatigue and tender cervical lymphadenopathy

PERITONSILLAR ABSCESS (QUINSY)

- Complication of tonsillitis
- Trismus and a "hot potato voice" should make you suspect a quinsy

PHARYNGEAL MALIGNANCY

- Persistent sore throat in older patients; smoking and alcohol excess are risk factors
- Weight loss, loss of appetite, fatigue, hard cervical lymphadenopathy and dysphagia
- Older patients diagnosed with tonsillitis should be followed up to ensure resolution

GASTRO-OESOPHAGEAL REFLUX

- Sore throat can be caused by reflux (which may otherwise be asymptomatic)
- Throat clearing, acid brash and a previous history of reflux are common features

DENTAL CAUSE OR MOUTH ULCERS

- If no medical cause is found, consider whether there could be a dental cause
- Dental abscesses usually present with localised pain around one tooth
- Trismus may be present

INVESTIGATIONS

- Examination of oropharynx is usually suffice to make a diagnosis
- If the cause is unclear despite this or red flags present consider acute referral
- Flexible nasoendoscopy to look for evidence of supraglottis or pharyngeal malignancy
- Bloods including FBC, LFTs and monospot to look for glandular fever (note: CRP is often raised to very high levels in streptococcal tonsillitis)

MANAGEMENT

- Analgesia – paracetamol, anti-inflammatories, benzydamine oral mouth rinse
- Consider oral antibiotics for tonsillitis, especially if CENTOR score is 3 or more
- Glandular fever – avoid contact sports for 6 weeks; rest; anti-pyretics
- Quinsy – Aspiration (secondary care) and IV antibiotics
- Pharyngeal malignancy – 2-week wait referral (surgery/chemotherapy/radiotherapy)
- Reflux – Protein pump inhibitor, gaviscon and lifestyle measures

FURTHER READING

NICE CKS on sore throat, http://cks.nice.org.uk/sore-throat-acute

Ophthalmology

9

PAINFUL RED EYE

INITIATING THE SESSION

- Greet the patient, ask an open question and screen for other problems

MEDICAL PERSPECTIVE

SEQUENCE OF EVENTS

- **Open question** – Can you tell me more about your painful/red eye?
- **Timeline** – How did it start? Was it sudden or did it gradually worsen? How has it progressed since then?

SYMPTOM ANALYSIS (SOCRATES)

- **Site** – Is it affecting both eyes or just one? The whole eye or just part of it?
- **Onset** – When did you first notice your eye was red and painful?
- **Character** – Can you describe the pain?
- **Radiation** – Do you feel the pain anywhere else? Does it give you a headache?
- **Associated symptoms** – *See systems review*
- **Timing** – Is the pain always there or does it come and go? *If intermittent,* how long does it last for? How often do you get the pain?
- **Exacerbating/relieving factors** – Does anything make the pain better or worse? Is the pain worse on moving your eyes? Is it worse in bright light? Can you recall any trauma to your eye or foreign object going into your eye?
- **Severity** – How bad is the pain on a scale of 1–10? Does it stop you sleeping?

SYSTEMS REVIEW

- **Vision** – Is your vision affected? *If so,* in what way? Is it blurry? Are you still able to read small print?
- **Discharge** – Has there been any discharge?
- **Pruritus** – Does your eye itch?

> **RED FLAGS**
>
> *Drop in visual acuity*
> *Pain interrupts sleep*
> *Symptom progression*
> *Contact lens use*
> *Trauma*

- **Xerophthalmia** – Do you have trouble with dryness?
- **Halos** – Do you see halos around bright lights?
- **Constitutional** – Have you had a fever or been feeling poorly recently?
- **RS** – Have you recently had a bad cough?
- **GIT** – Do you have any trouble with your bowels? Abdominal pain? Any vomiting?
- **GUT** – Any urinary symptoms such as burning when passing urine or discharge? Have you been treated for any STIs?
- **MS** – Any pain in any joints? Do you have any rashes?

PATIENT'S PERSPECTIVE

- **Feelings and effect on life** – How have your symptoms affected you?
- **Ideas** – Do you have any ideas yourself about what could be causing the pain?
- **Concerns** – Is there anything you are particularly concerned could be causing it? Is there anything in general that concerns you?
- **Expectations** – Was there anything in particular you were hoping for when you made the appointment for today?

BACKGROUND INFORMATION

PMH

- Do you suffer from any medical conditions? Have you had trouble with your eyes in the past?
- Do you wear glasses or have a refractive error? *Long-sighted people are at an increased risk of angle closure glaucoma*
- *Ask specifically about inflammatory arthritis and IBD (HLA-B27-positive patients have a significant risk of anterior uveitis and scleritis)*

DH

- Do you take any medications? Do you have any allergies?
- *Ask specifically about systemic/topical steroids and topical eye drops*
- *Allergic conjunctivitis occurs in people who suffer with atopy such as hay fever*

FH

- Does anyone in the family suffer with eye problems, both recent and old?

SH

- Are you currently working? *If so*, what is your job? What does that involve? *Is there a high risk of a foreign body? (E.g. blacksmiths, engineers or manual labourers)*
- Can you tell me about your home situation (*occupants and any difficulties*)?
- Has your problem affected your job or home life in any way?
- Do you wear contact lenses? (*Poor lens hygiene can cause microbial keratitis*)

CLOSING THE SESSION

- summary ± examination/explanation and planning/contract

IMPORTANT POINTS

- A red eye may be obvious, but eye pain can be misleading – If pain is the only symptom, you may need to think laterally e.g. could this be a cluster headache or other non-ophthalmological issue with referred pain? Similarly, patients may present with what is thought to be a headache or subarachnoid haemorrhage, only to have their red eye neglected

DIFFERENTIAL DIAGNOSIS

Although the acute red eye is a common complaint and often entirely benign, it can also represent an acute ocular emergency which requires rapid evaluation and treatment in order to preserve vision. It is therefore important to be able to identify the serious diagnoses so that the appropriate action can be taken, if needed, to prevent permanent damage to vision.

CONJUNCTIVITIS (VIRAL, BACTERIAL, ALLERGIC); (MOST COMMON)

- Usually unilateral, but later may become bilateral due to autoinoculation
- Conjuctival injection (red sclera), watery or purulent discharge
- Allergic – Abrupt onset after exposure, bilateral, with chemosis, pruritus and eyelid oedema; watery discharge with foreign body sensation, nasal congestion and hives may also be present; tends to have seasonal variation

ACUTE ANGLE CLOSURE GLAUCOMA (MOST SERIOUS)

- Ophthalmological emergency – If not treated rapidly, will result in irreversible damage to the optic nerve and retina from pressure-induced ischaemia
- Presents unilaterally, commonly in the evening due to low light levels causing a mid-dilated pupil increasing the risk of angle closure
- Symptoms include red eye, pain (globe, headache and abdominal), blurred vision, haloes around lights and nausea and vomiting

INFECTIOUS KERATITIS (BACTERIAL, FUNGAL, PARASITIC, HERPES SIMPLEX, HERPES ZOSTER)

- Unilaterally painful eye that mimics conjunctivitis
- There is a foreign body sensation, photophobia and reduced vision
- Bacterial keratitis is much more likely in contact lens wearers or the immunocompromised
- Potentially blinding due to corneal scarring and neovascularisation or perforation – Therefore warrants immediate ophthalmological referral

ACUTE ANTERIOR UVEITIS

- Acute pain, often a recurring event, in one eye with associated photophobia, redness and blurred vision
- Typically, the pain is felt more deeply than in conjunctivitis
- *Photophobia occurs because the iris is inflamed and so miosis is painful*
- There may be a background history of HLA-B27-associated spondyloarthropathies, IBD, Reiter's syndrome and/or psoriasis

EPISCLERITIS

- Injection of a localised area or diffuse area overlying the sclera with a non-tender globe
- Often recurrent and characterised by rapid onset of a dull ache, redness and tenderness
- Vision not effected

SCLERITIS

- Severely painful, sub-acute onset with associated tearing and photophobia
- Tender globe to touch, painful eye movements
- Often recurrent and bilateral, though not simultaneously
- Strongly associated with rheumatoid arthritis, ANCA-positive vasculitis and SLE
- Potentially sight threatening, may result in astigmatism

SUBCONJUNCTIVAL HAEMORRHAGE

- Diffusely red eye unilaterally with no associated pain or visual disturbance
- Often after an episode of coughing, vomiting or straining
- May be caused by trauma – Exclude globe damage or foreign body
- Resolves spontaneously

INVESTIGATIONS

- Thorough eye examination, including visual fields
- Dilated ophthalmoscopy, ideally a slit lamp examination (do not dilate if you suspect angle closure)
- Tonometry
- Conjunctival and corneal swabs/scrape for culture/PCR
- Syphilis serology, chest x-ray and HLA-B27 testing for complex uveitis
- Gonioscopy

MANAGEMENT

- Acute angle closure – IV acetazolamide, dexamethasone, pilocarpine, timolol and iopidine, all immediately; peripheral iridotomy
- Viral conjunctivitis – Cool compress for symptomatic relief
- Bacterial conjunctivitis – Topical chloramphenicol
- Allergic conjunctivitis – Topical mast cell stabilisers for prophylaxis; topical antihistamines for symptomatic relief; oral steroids for severe disease
- Herpes simplex keratitis – Topical aciclovir
- Herpes zoster ophthalmicus – Oral aciclovir
- Anterior uveitis – Cycloplegia for symptomatic relief; topical steroid to induce remission

FURTHER READING

NICE CKS on the red eye, http://cks.nice.org.uk/red-eye

LOSS OF VISION/BLURRY VISION

INITIATING THE SESSION

- Greet the patient, ask an open question and screen for other problems

MEDICAL PERSPECTIVE

SEQUENCE OF EVENTS

- **Open question** – Can you tell me more about the problems with your vision?
- **Timeline** – How did it start? Was it sudden or did it gradually worsen? Was it like a curtain coming down? How has it progressed since then?

SYMPTOM ANALYSIS

- **Clarify** – What exactly do you mean by loss of vision? Is your vision blurry or are you missing parts of your vision? *If blurry,* do you see double or is it just all unclear? *If double vision,* are the images side-by-side or one above the other? Does it go away if you occlude one eye?
- **Site** – Is this in both eyes or one eye only? Is it in the entire eye or part of it? Which part of your vision is missing/affected? Left or right? Upper or lower vision? Do you have tunnel vision?
- **Central vision** – Is the centre of your vision affected when you look directly at something?
- **Colour vision** – Have you noticed a change in your colour vision?
- **Remaining vision** – How much vision remains? Are you able to recognise faces, read small text or see any light?
- **Triggers** – Did anything precipitate this? Any history of trauma?

SYSTEMS REVIEW

- **Pain** – Do you have any pain in your eyes or around your eyes? Is it painful to move your eyes? Any headache?
- **Injection** – Have you noticed any redness in your eyes?
- **Flashes and floaters** – Have you noticed any flashes of light or floaters?
- **NS** – Have you seen any zig-zag lines? Do you have any weakness or pins and needles? Have you had any trouble with your speech?
- **Hypertension** – Do you get any morning headaches on waking?
- **Temporal arteritis** – Do you get a cramping pain in your jaw when chewing food? Is it painful to comb your hair?

> **RED FLAGS**
>
> *Profound loss of vision*
> *Rapid onset*
> *Pain*
> *Trauma*

PATIENT'S PERSPECTIVE

- **Feelings and effect on life** – How has your change in vision affected you?
- **Ideas** – Do you have any ideas yourself about what could be causing it?
- **Concerns** – Is there anything you are particularly concerned could be causing it? Is there anything in general that concerns you?
- **Expectations** – Was there anything in particular you were hoping for when you made the appointment for today?

BACKGROUND INFORMATION

PMH

- Do you suffer from any medical conditions?
- *Ask specifically about diabetes, hypertension and atrial fibrillation*
- Have you ever had any trouble with your eyes in the past? Do you suffer from short sightedness? Do you see an ophthalmologist regularly or for screening?

DH

- Have you recently started taking any new medications? Do you have any allergies?
- *Ask specifically about digoxin*

FH

- Does anyone in the family have trouble with their vision?
- *Ask specifically about glaucoma and retinitis pigmentosa*

SH

- Are you currently working? *If so,* what is your job? What does that involve?
- Can you tell me about your home situation (*occupants and any difficulties*)?
- Do you drive?
- Has your problem affected your job or home life in any way?
- Do you smoke? Do you drink alcohol? Do you drink homemade alcohol?
- Do you take any illicit drugs or inject yourself?

CLOSING THE SESSION

- summary ± examination/explanation and planning/contract

IMPORTANT POINTS

- Beware patients with homonymous defects may report monocular blindness when they mean one side of their visual field is missing
- Some patients fail to notice a monocular blindness until their good eye is covered!
- Some drugs have been known to cause sudden disturbance in vision. E.g. digoxin can cause the vision to become more yellowish
- IV drug abuse may result in septic emboli in the retinal vessels
- Moonshine and antifreeze have been known to cause toxic optic neuropathy, whilst B12 deficiency in alcoholism can result in optic atrophy
- Very important that the patient's ability to drive is approached. It is the patient's responsibility to inform the DVLA

DIFFERENTIAL DIAGNOSIS

An instant change in vision is more likely to be due to vascular occlusion. A horizontal defect suggests a retinal vascular cause, whereas a vertical defect suggests a neuro-ophthalmic problem.

ACUTE VISUAL LOSS

RETINAL ARTERY OCCLUSION

- Sudden onset of persistent monocular visual loss
- Exact field defect dependant on whether it is a central or branch occlusion (branch occlusion will produce a horizontal field loss)
- Amaurosis fugax, hypercoagulable state and atherosclerotic risk factors may be present

RETINAL VEIN OCCLUSION

- Acute painless monocular mild to moderate visual loss

TEMPORAL ARTERITIS

- May present as a recent severe headache over the temporal region
- Jaw claudication, scalp tenderness and proximal muscle stiffness and aching
- Transient/permanent visual loss, blurred vision and amaurosis fugax
- Patients >55 y/o and if left untreated, will affect the other eye in weeks

OPTIC NEURITIS

- Often young female patients and may be first presentation of multiple sclerosis
- Deep pain associated with eye movements and a central scotoma
- Symptoms exacerbated by raising body temperature (e.g. exercise/hot baths)
- Neurological symptoms such as weakness or paraesthesia

RETINAL DETACHMENT

- Signs and symptoms include flashes of light, floaters and a peripheral scotoma
- Risk factors include myopia (thin retina), recent cataract surgery and diabetes

VITREOUS DETACHMENT

- Common cause of acute visual disturbance, affecting the middle aged/elderly
- Chronic floaters, with a sudden increase in the number of floaters and possibly flashing lights as the vitreous starts to pull away from the retina
- May result in retinal detachment or vitreal haemorrhage
- Visual acuity not affected and usually self-limiting

VITREOUS HAEMORRHAGE

- Spontaneous bleeding from the retinal vessels into the vitreous
- Sudden onset of altered vision, blobs and floaters
- Visual acuity is variable depending on site and size of haemorrhage

CEREBRAL VASCULAR ACCIDENT

- Sudden onset of homonymous visual field defect
- Patient may describe it as losing vision in one eye when in fact it is the entire left or right visual field that has gone
- Weakness, paraesthesia, dysphasia and ataxia may also be present

GRADUAL VISUAL LOSS

GLAUCOMA

- Usually asymptomatic; may develop visual field loss with negative scotomas typically found in the nasal field
- Blurring and haloes around lights may occur due to corneal oedema
- Risk factors include Afro-Caribbean ethnicity, diabetes, advanced age, myopia and family history

CATARACT

- History of blurred vision, glare from bright lights, increasing myopia, yellowish/brown discolouration, monocular diplopia and poor night vision
- Gradual worsening of symptoms
- Risk factors include advancing age and diabetes

MACULAR DEGENERATION

- Gradual onset of worsening visual acuity and a central scotoma
- Metamorphopsia, where images become distorted is also a common complaint

RETINITIS PIGMENTOSA

- Nyctalopia, decreased visual acuity and loss of peripheral vision
- Nearly 50% is inherited in autosomal dominant, recessive or x-linked pattern

OPTIC NEUROPATHY

- Multiple causes. If caused by compressive lesion, may have occulomotility defect or isolated visual field defect
- Nutritional or toxic optic neuropathy caused by excessive alcohol, smoking or diet deficient in vitamin B12
- Can be inherited. Consider if strong family history of visual loss

INVESTIGATIONS

- Eye examination, including visual fields, acuity and ophthalmoscopy
- ESR and temporal artery biopsy if suspecting temporal arteritis
- Ocular coherence topography
- Fundus fluorescein angiography if wet AMD is suspected

- USS of posterior segment
- Tonometry and pachymetry where glaucoma is suspected
- Visual fields
- Carotid doppler and echocardiogram for source of emboli
- MRI for diagnosis of multiple sclerosis
- Electro-physiology for optic neuropathy of unknown cause

MANAGEMENT

- **Retinal artery occlusion** – Ocular massage may help improve outcome
- **Retinal vein occlusion** – Lifestyle factors (smoking cessation, blood pressure control and diabetic control); ischaemic retinal vein occlusion – Pan-retinal photocoagulation and anti-VEGF antibodies
- **Temporal arteritis** – High-dose oral steroids
- **Optic neuritis** – IV and oral steroids can hasten recovery of optic neuritis but not improve final vision
- **Retinal detachment** – Surgical repair
- **Macular degeneration (wet)** – Intravitreal anti-VEGF therapy
- **Retinitis pigmentosa** – Vitamin A to slow progression
- **Cataracts** – Phacoemulsification and implantation of a prosthetic lens

FURTHER READING

NICE CKS on:

Glaucoma, http://cks.nice.org.uk/glaucoma
Cataracts, http://cks.nice.org.uk/cataracts
Retinal detachment, http://cks.nice.org.uk/retinal-detachment
Temporal arteritis, http://cks.nice.org.uk/giant-cell-arteritis

Obstetrics and gynaecology

10

GYNAECOLOGICAL HISTORY TEMPLATE

For the general gynaecological history, the following components should be considered as part of the review. These are referred to in the subsequent histories in this section.

MENSTRUAL HISTORY

- Is there any chance you could be pregnant? How have your periods been?
- **Last menstrual period** – When was the first day of your last period?
- **Cycle** – Are your periods regular every so many days? How often are your periods (*in days*)? How long do they usually last for?
- **Menarche** – What age were you when you had your first period?
- **Menorrhagia** – Do you suffer from heavy or painful periods?
- *If menopausal, establish whether they are taking hormone replacement therapy*

VAGINAL BLEEDING (SOCRAT)

- **Site** – Where is the bleeding coming from? Is it definitely coming from the vagina?
- **Onset** – When did you first notice it?
- **Character** – How much have you noticed? Have you passed clots? What colour is it?
- **Radiation** – Do you use tampons or padding? Does it soak them?
- **Associated symptoms** – *Pain, discharge, menstruation and constitutional symptoms*
- **Timing** – When do you notice the bleeding? Is it there all the time? How often have you noticed it? Could it be your period? Does it occur mid-cycle? Does it come on after sex?

PAIN

- **Abdominal pain** – Do you have any pain in your abdomen or further down?
- **Dyspareunia** – Have you had any pain during sex? *If so,* where exactly? Is it a deep pain or a more superficial pain on entering?

VAGINAL DISCHARGE (*ALSO RELEVANT FOR PENILE DISCHARGE*)

- Have you noticed any discharge? Can you tell me about the discharge?
- **Colour** – What colour is the discharge?
- **Odour** – Does it have a particularly bad smell? *If so,* is it fishy smelling?
- **Amount** – How much have you noticed?

SEXUAL HISTORY

- **Last cervical smear** – When was your last smear done?
- **Sexually active** – Are you sexually active?
- **Partner(s)** – Is it with a regular partner or different partners?
- **Contraception/HRT** – Are you currently taking contraception/hormone replacement therapy? *Specify and check compliance*
- *Take a history of sexual encounters if relevant (e.g. discharge present)*

OBSTETRIC HISTORY

- **Gravida** – Is this your first pregnancy? *Take history of each pregnancy in chronological order*
- **Complications** – Have you had any complications during any of the pregnancies? Have you suffered any miscarriages, stillbirths or terminations?
- **Gestational age** – How many weeks' gestation was your baby at delivery?
- **Delivery** – How was he/she delivered? *If by caesarean section,* why was this needed?
- **Birth weight** – What was his/her birth weight?

VAGINAL BLEEDING

INITIATING THE SESSION

- Greet the patient, ask an open question and screen for other problems

MEDICAL PERSPECTIVE

SEQUENCE OF EVENTS

- **Open question** – Can you tell me more about the bleeding?
- **Timeline** – How did it start? How has it progressed since then?

SYMPTOM ANALYSIS (SOCRAT)

- **Site** – When and where exactly did you notice the bleeding? Is it definitely coming from the vagina?
- **Onset** – When did you first notice it?
- **Character** – How much have you noticed? Have you passed clots? What colour is it?
- **Radiation** – Do you use tampons or padding? Does it soak them?
- **Associated symptoms** – *See systems review*
- **Timing** – When do you notice the bleeding? Is it there all the time? How often have you noticed it? Could it be your period? Does it occur mid-cycle? Does it come on after sex?

SYSTEMS REVIEW (*SEE GYNAECOLOGICAL HISTORY TEMPLATE*)

- **Menstrual history**
- **Pain**
- **Sexual history**
- **Vaginal discharge**
- **Obstetric history**
- **Constitutional** – Have you felt feverish? Any weight loss? How is your appetite? Have you been particularly tired recently? Have you been breathless at all?

> **RED FLAGS**
>
> *Severe pain*
> *5–12 weeks since LMP*
> *Weight loss*
> *Postmenopausal bleeding*
> *Intermenstrual bleeding*
> *Postcoital bleeding*
> *Missed cervical smears*

PATIENT'S PERSPECTIVE

- **Feelings and effect on life** – How have your symptoms affected your daily life?
- **Ideas** – Do you have any ideas yourself about what could be causing the bleeding?
- **Concerns** – Is there anything you are particularly concerned could be causing it? Is there anything in general that concerns you?
- **Expectations** – Was there anything in particular you were hoping for when you made the appointment for today?

BACKGROUND INFORMATION

PMH

- Do you suffer from any medical conditions?
- *Ask specifically about previous cancer (particularly breast, ovarian, endometrial and cervical), STIs and bleeding disorders*

DH

- Are you currently taking any medication? Do you have any allergies?

FH

- Do any conditions run in the family?
- *Ask about breast and ovarian cancer; determine in whom and when they were diagnosed*

SH

- Are you currently working?
- Do you smoke? Drink alcohol? How much?
- Are you currently working? *If so*, what is your job? What does that involve?
- Can you tell me about your home situation (*occupants and any difficulties*)?
- Has your problem affected your job or home life in any way?

CLOSING THE SESSION

- summary ± examination/explanation and planning/contract

IMPORTANT POINTS

- This is often an embarrassing complaint for patients, so use tact and try ways to make the patient feel more comfortable talking to you. E.g. "Often people feel embarrassed talking about this, but it is a common issue. I am here to help and I will keep everything we talk about strictly confidential"
- It is extremely important to ask when their last cervical smear was performed, as well as considering constitutional symptoms, to show you are thinking about cervical and endometrial cancer as possible diagnoses
- Enquiring about contraceptive method(s) used and compliance is important to help establish the correct diagnosis. Condoms used regularly decrease the likelihood of cervical cancer; hormonal contraception may suggest breakthrough bleeding; whilst intra-uterine contraceptive devices increase the risk of ectopic pregnancy
- You must also establish whether there is a chance the patient could be pregnant as this might point to a very different diagnosis (e.g. ectopic pregnancy)

DIFFERENTIAL DIAGNOSIS

Differential diagnosis of a PV bleed depends on the timing of the bleed – menstrual, inter-menstrual, postcoital or postmenopausal. Heavy menstrual bleeding is known as menorrhagia. Do they have a bleeding disorder, or are they on anti-coagulants?

POSTCOITAL

CERVICAL CARCINOMA

- Infection with human papillomavirus (HPV) 16 and 18
- History of multiple partners, STIs, smoking, missed smears, weight loss and loss of appetite
- Can also present as intermenstrual bleeding

CERVICAL ECTROPION

- Squamocolumnar junction extends under hormonal influence (e.g. puberty, COCP and pregnancy)
- Red ring around cervical os on examination with speculum

CERVICAL POLYP

- May bleed on contact
- Can also present as intermenstrual bleeding

POSTMENOPAUSAL (PV BLEEDING >12 MONTHS AFTER LAST PERIOD)

ENDOMETRIAL CARCINOMA

- Risk factors – Unopposed oestrogen exposure, obesity, old age, nulliparity, late menopause and polycystic ovarian syndrome
- Accounts for ~10% of postmenopausal bleeding but requires urgent investigation
- Less commonly can present as postcoital or intermenstrual bleeding

ATROPHIC VAGINITIS

- Dry, itchy vagina with subsequent dyspareunia
- Urinary incontinence and recurrent UTIs
- Very common in postmenopausal women due to low levels of oestrogen

ENDOMETRIAL HYPERPLASIA

- Exposure to high levels of oestrogen with insufficient levels of progesterone
- Diagnosed on endometrial biopsy or curettage
- Significant risk factor for development of endometrial carcinoma

INTERMENSTRUAL

Some women experience light bleeding or spotting that is normal during ovulation (~day 14 of cycle). Always consider if the patient could be pregnant. Spotting may occur with implantation of the blastocyst in the uterus but also with conditions associated with pregnancy. Breakthrough bleeding is also common in the first few months of starting a hormonal contraception.

ECTOPIC PREGNANCY

- Severe, sharp, colicky abdominal pain in a sexually active woman
- Diarrhoea and vomiting may also be present
- Rupture leads to severe pain, peritonism and shock
- Occurs ~5–12 weeks after last period
- Occurs due to fertilised ovum implanting outside uterine cavity
- Increased risk of ectopic pregnancy if using intrauterine contraceptive device

SPONTANEOUS ABORTION

- Loss of pregnancy at any stage up to the 24th week
- Lower abdominal cramps, passing blood clots with "tissue"

SEXUALLY TRANSMITTED INFECTION

- Sexually active woman with discharge that may be smelly
- Risk factors – Young/adolescent, multiple partners/new partner, unprotected sex

INVESTIGATIONS

- Abdominal and pelvic examination – feel for any pelvic masses
- PV Examination – Confirm it is a PV bleed; look for pathology
- Bloods – FBC and clotting
- Urine beta-hCG (pregnancy test)
- STI screen – high vaginal and endocervical swabs
- Cervical smear (if due/overdue for smear)
- Colposcopy after abnormal smear
- Transvaginal USS
- Urgent USS if suspect ectopic pregnancy

MANAGEMENT

- Urgent referral for PMB or IMB/PCB if suspicion arises from PV exam
- **Atrophic vaginitis** – Topical lubricant/cream or HRT (topical or systemic)
- **Polyps** – Remove and send for histology
- **Ectopic pregnancy** – Surgical intervention (either laparoscopic or open)
- **STI** – Appropriate antibiotic treatment

FURTHER READING

NICE CKS on:
> Menorrhagia, http://cks.nice.org.uk/menorrhagia
> Cancers, http://cks.nice.org.uk/gynaecological-cancers-recognition-and-referral

Patient.co.uk professional article on irregular per vaginal bleeding, http://patient.info/doctor/intermenstrual-and-postcoital-bleeding

ANTEPARTUM HAEMORRHAGE

INITIATING THE SESSION

- Greet the patient, ask an open question and screen for other problems

MEDICAL PERSPECTIVE

SEQUENCE OF EVENTS

- **Open question** – Can you tell me more about the bleeding?
- **Timeline** – How did it start? How has it progressed since then?

SYMPTOM ANALYSIS (SOCRAT)

- **Site** – When and where exactly did you notice the bleeding? Is it definitely coming from the vagina?
- **Onset** – When did you first notice the bleeding?
- **Character** – How much have you noticed? What colour is it? Have you passed clots or anything odd?
- **Radiation** – Have you had to use padding? Does it soak them?
- **Associated symptoms** – *See systems review*
- **Timing** – Is the bleeding there all the time? How often have you noticed it?

CURRENT PREGNANCY

- **Foetal well-being** – Have you felt the baby moving recently? Have you had any pain down below or in your tummy?
- **Last menstrual period** – When was the first day of your last period?
- **Progress** – How has the pregnancy gone previously to this? Have you been suffering from high blood pressure, water infections or anything else?
- **Tests** – What tests been performed so far?

SYSTEMS REVIEW (*SEE GYNAECOLOGICAL HISTORY TEMPLATE*)

- **Pain**
- **Obstetric history**

PATIENT'S PERSPECTIVE

- **Feelings and effect on life** – I appreciate this can be very distressing. How has this made you feel? What effect has this had on you?
- **Ideas** – Do you have any ideas yourself about what could be causing the bleeding?
- **Concerns** – Is there anything you are particularly concerned could be causing it? Is there anything in general that concerns you?
- **Expectations** – Was there anything in particular you were hoping for when you made the appointment for today?

> **RED FLAGS**
>
> *Severe pain*
> *Large volume blood loss*
> *Multiparity*
> *Previous caesarian section(s)*
> *Advanced maternal age*
> *Previous antepartum haemorrhage*

BACKGROUND INFORMATION

PMH

- Do you suffer from any medical conditions?
- *Ask specifically about bleeding disorders, lupus (antiphospholipid syndrome predisposes to recurrent miscarriages), hypertension and diabetes*

DH

- Are you taking any medications? (*Are any of them contraindicated in pregnancy?*)
- Do you have any allergies?

FH

- Do any conditions run in your family?
- Has anyone in your family had problems during pregnancies?

SH

- Do you smoke? Drink alcohol? How much? Do you take any recreational drugs?
- *If answered yes to any of the above* – Have you stopped since you found out you were pregnant? Are you aware of the problems continuing to do so can have to your child?
- Are you currently working? *If so,* what is your job? What does that involve?
- Can you tell me about your home situation (*occupants and any difficulties*)?
- Has your problem affected your job or home life in any way? Who is there to support you?

CLOSING THE SESSION

- summary ± examination/explanation and planning/contract

IMPORTANT POINTS

- Read the instructions outside the station carefully – Does it only ask you to take a history? You may be required not only to take a history but also to examine the patient, give your diagnosis and determine your investigations and management
- Consider at the start whether or not the patient is well enough to take a history from; if the patient is critically unwell, then an ABCDE approach should be initiated ASAP and the history should be sought later
- If the patient is haemodynamically stable, but you suspect urgent assessment is needed, consider taking a shortened history of the symptoms and then move on to examination and investigations

DIFFERENTIAL DIAGNOSIS

Antepartum haemorrhage includes any genital bleeding from the 24th week of gestation up to term. In many cases, the cause of antepartum haemorrhage is of undetermined origin

PLACENTAL ABRUPTION (MOST SERIOUS)

- Placenta either partially or completely detaches from uterus
- Painful bleeding with foetal distress
- Bleeding may be concealed and therefore not appear as severe as it actually is
- Risk factors include smoking, trauma, previous abruption and multiparity

PLACENTA PRAEVIA

- Placenta lying in the lower uterine segment; often found incidentally by USS
- Intermittent painless bleeding of increasing intensity and frequency
- Foetal distress is not common but can occur with complications of praevia
- Risk factors include previous smoking, increasing age and obstetric complications such as previous praevia, miscarriage and spontaneous abortion

NON-PREGNANCY-RELATED CAUSES

CERVICAL ECTROPION (MOST COMMON)

- Common in pregnancy
- Red ring around cervical os on examination with speculum

CERVICAL POLYP

- Bleeding may occur postcoitally (contact bleeding) or anytime

CERVICAL CANCER

- Bleeding may occur postcoitally (contact bleeding) or anytime
- History of multiple partners, STIs, smoking, missed smears, weight loss, loss of appetite

INVESTIGATIONS

- An ABCDE approach should be used if the patient is acutely unwell (airways, breathing, circulation, disability and exposure) – In this case, resuscitating the patient is the primary objective; the patient should be admitted to hospital
- Bloods – FBC, cross-match and clotting
- Must not perform vaginal examination unless placenta praevia excluded by USS as massive haemorrhage may be provoked
- Antenatal examination – Breech presentation with transverse lie common in praevia
- Pelvic USS
- Cardiotocography – Evidence of foetal distress? Monitor foetal well-being

MANAGEMENT

- If required, resuscitation (100% oxygen, large bore cannulae and fluids)
- Give analgesia if needed

- Prophylactic anti-D immunoglobulin for rhesus negative women
- Admission until delivery by caesarean section at 39 weeks or praevia
- Urgent caesarean section if foetal distress or severe bleeding

FURTHER READING

Royal College of Obstetrics and Gynaecology guidance on antepartum haemorrhage, https://www.rcog.org.uk/globalassets/documents/guidelines/gtg63_05122011aph.pdf

VAGINAL DISCHARGE

INITIATING THE SESSION

- Greet the patient, ask an open question and screen for other problems

MEDICAL PERSPECTIVE

SEQUENCE OF EVENTS

- **Open question** – Can you tell me more about the discharge?
- **Timeline** – How did it start? How has it progressed since then?

SYMPTOM ANALYSIS

- **Onset** – When did you first notice it?
- **Colour** – What colour is it? Is there any blood?
- **Odour** – Does it have a particularly bad or distinctive smell?
- **Amount** – How much discharge have you noticed?

SYSTEMS REVIEW (*SEE GYNAECOLOGICAL HISTORY TEMPLATE*)

- **Pain**
- **Menstrual history**
- **Sexual history**

PATIENT'S PERSPECTIVE

- **Feelings and effect on life** – How have your symptoms affected your daily life?
- **Ideas** – Do you have any ideas yourself about what could be causing the discharge?
- **Concerns** – Is there anything you are particularly concerned could be causing it? Is there anything in general that concerns you?
- **Expectations** – Was there anything in particular you were hoping for when you made the appointment for today?

BACKGROUND INFORMATION

PMH

- Do you suffer from any medical conditions?
- Have you ever had an STI? *If so, specify which one, when, how it was treated and whether the partner(s) was also treated*

DH

- Are you taking any medications? Do you have any allergies?

FH

- Do any conditions run in the family?

SH

- Do you drink alcohol? Smoke? How much? Do you take any recreational drugs?
- Are you currently working? *If so,* what is your job? What does that involve?
- Can you tell me about your home situation (*occupants and any difficulties*)?
- Has your problem affected your job or home life in any way?

CLOSING THE SESSION

- summary ± examination/explanation and planning/contract

IMPORTANT POINTS

- Stress confidentiality aspect to patient
- Non-judgemental approach throughout history is obviously imperative
- Prepare grounds for sexual history before beginning that aspect
- In the sexual history, start with the least intrusive questions and gradually work your way to the potentially most embarrassing ones
- Never take a sexual history in parallel – one partner at a time only
- See patient alone – partners, family or friends may prevent the patient from revealing personal information
- Do not make assumptions about sexual orientation and relationships – use neutral terms such as "partner"
- Remember STIs "hunt in packs." If they have one STI they may well have another
- Never forget to ask when their last smear was performed – cervical cancer is strongly linked with human papilloma virus infection which is passed on sexually

---

DIFFERENTIAL DIAGNOSIS

PHYSIOLOGICAL DISCHARGE (NORMAL)

- Clear/creamy, thin and stringy discharge
- Amount varies but typically increases with pregnancy, COCP, around ovulation and during sexual arousal

SEXUALLY TRANSMITTED INFECTION

- *Chlamydia trachomatis* – Although asymptomatic in the majority of women, chlamydia can cause copious purulent discharge and dysuria
- *Trichomonas vaginalis* – Copious amounts of green/yellow discharge that may smell fishy
- *Neisseria gonorrhoea* – Often asymptomatic in women but can cause purulent discharge
- HIV, syphilis, genital herpes and genital warts are not associated with vaginal discharge themselves, although as STIs "hunt in packs," discharge is likely to be present in these cases as well

NON-SEXUALLY TRANSMITTED INFECTION

- Vulvovaginal candidiasis (thrush) – Thick, white "cottage cheese" discharge, with an itchy, red and tender vagina; associated with pregnancy, COCP, antibiotics and immunodeficiency

- Bacterial vaginosis – Grey-white, fishy-smelling discharge predisposed to by increasing vaginal pH levels (e.g. by sperm, menstruation or using soaps), which kills protective lactobacilli

PELVIC INFLAMMATORY DISEASE

- Abdominal/pelvic pain, dyspareunia and abnormal vaginal bleeding may also occur
- May be asymptomatic, presenting later as subfertility or a menstrual disorder
- History of previously known STIs may not be present as could be asymptomatic

FOREIGN BODY

- Most commonly forgetting to remove a tampon after menstruation
- Foul smelling
- Can result in toxic shock syndrome

GENITAL TRACT MALIGNANCY

- Red/brown discharge (blood) likely to be smelly

INVESTIGATIONS

- Pelvic examination to look for structural abnormalities, presence of foreign bodies and cervical excitation (for pelvic inflammatory disease)
- High vaginal swab for bacterial vaginosis, candida, trichomonas and gonorrhoea
- Endocervical swabs for gonorrhoea (culture) and chlamydia (PCR analysis)
- Cervical smear test if not already performed under Cervical Screening Programme
- Same day referral to GUM clinic for suspected pelvic inflammatory disease or admit if systemically unwell
- Urgent referral for any patient with suspicion of a genital tract malignancy

MANAGEMENT

- Removal of foreign bodies to prevent toxic shock syndrome
- All patients with confirmed STIs should ideally be referred to the GUM clinic for treatment and contact tracing
- Trichomonas and bacterial vaginosis – Metronidazole 7-day course
- Vulvovaginal candidiasis – Clotrimazole pessary or oral fluconazole stat dose
- Chlamydia – Stat dose of azithromycin or 7-day course of doxycycline
- Gonorrhoea – Stat dose of oral cefixime or IM ceftriaxone and oral azithromycin
- Pelvic inflammatory disease – 14-day course of metronidazole and ofloxacin ± stat dose of IM ceftriaxone
- Abstinence from sex until treatment completed for patient and partner(s)

FURTHER READING

NICE CKS on vaginal discharge, http://cks.nice.org.uk/vaginal-discharge

SUBFERTILITY

INITIATING THE SESSION

- Greet the patient, ask an open question and screen for other problems

MEDICAL PERSPECTIVE

SEQUENCE OF EVENTS AND SYMPTOM ANALYSIS (*CHECK BOTH PARTNERS' RESPONSES*)

- **Open question** – Can you tell me more about the problem?
- **Duration** – How long have you been trying for a baby?
- **Regular sex** – Do you have regular sex? How often?
- **Type of sex** – Can I just check that you mean penetrative vaginal sexual intercourse?
- **Problems** – Do either of you have any problems having sex? Any pain during sex? Any bleeding after sex? Are there any anxieties or fears around sex? (*this question is best asked with each partner one-to-one where possible*)

SYSTEM'S REVIEW (*SEE GYNAECOLOGICAL HISTORY TEMPLATE*)

- **Menstrual history**
- **Obstetric history** (*including any previous pregnancies*)

PATIENT'S PERSPECTIVE

- **Feelings and effect on life** – Has everything you mentioned had an impact on you mentally or in daily life? How is your mood?
- **Ideas** – Do you have any idea about why you may be having difficulty conceiving?
- **Concerns** – Is there anything you are particularly concerned could be causing it? Is there anything in general that concerns you?
- **Expectations** – Was there anything in particular you were hoping for when you made the appointment for today?

BACKGROUND INFORMATION (*CHECK BOTH PARTNERS' RESPONSES UNLESS INDICATED OTHERWISE*)

PMH

- Have you ever suffered from any medical conditions?
- *Ask the woman about miscarriages, polycystic ovarian syndrome, STIs, gynaecological surgery and previous cancer (including chemotherapy and radiotherapy)*
- *Ask the man about mumps, STIs, testicular torsion, vasectomy, trauma and previous cancer (including chemotherapy and radiotherapy)*

DH

- Are you currently taking any medications? Do you have any allergies?
- Have you tried taking any medications to assist conception previously?
- What contraception have you used in the past? *Take full details*

FH

- Has anyone in your family had difficulty in conceiving a child?

SH

- Are you currently working? *If so,* what is your job? What does that involve? Do you spend long periods away from your partner?
- Can you tell me about your home situation (*occupants and any difficulties*)?
- Has your problem affected your job or home life in any way?
- Do you smoke? Do you drink alcohol? Have you ever taken any recreational drugs?
- I know this is a personal question, but can I ask how much you weigh?

CLOSING THE SESSION

- summary ± examination/explanation and planning/contract

IMPORTANT POINTS

- In any history regarding a couple's difficulty conceiving, it is extremely important that both partners are present and that questions are directed at both of them as the problem could lie with either one.
- This can be a sensitive history and often the best way to approach it is to be direct and not appear informal or uncomfortable yourself when conducting the interview

DIFFERENTIAL DIAGNOSIS

The cause of subfertility can be due to problems with the male, female or both. In many couples the cause is unexplained, of whom many will conceive at a later date.

GENERAL CAUSES

- Not having regular satisfactory penetrative sexual intercourse
  - Dyspareunia
  - Psychosexual issues
  - Partner away for large periods of time
  - Premature ejaculation before penetration achieved
- Recreational drugs, alcohol and smoking can all impair fertility

FEMALE CAUSES

- Age – Female fertility tends to decrease after mid-30s
- Being overweight (or markedly underweight)

- Systemic conditions e.g. SLE
- Iatrogenic causes e.g. pelvic surgery or chemotherapy
- Ovulatory disorders
  - Polycystic ovarian syndrome
  - Hyperprolactinaemia
  - Thyroid disorders
  - Premature menopause
  - Hypogonadotrophic hypogonadism
- Tubal pathology
  - Pelvic inflammatory disease
  - Endometriosis
- Uterine pathology
  - Fibroids
  - Uterine abnormalities

MALE CAUSES

- Testicular trauma
- Testicular torsion
- Bilateral undescended testicles
- Systemic conditions
- Chemotherapy
- Mumps with orchitis
- Gonorrhoea and chlamydia
- Retrograde ejaculation after transurethral resection of the prostate

INVESTIGATIONS

- Abdominal and bimanual examination
  - Uterine abnormalities
  - Ovarian cysts
  - Cervical excitation for possible pelvic inflammatory disease
  - Vaginismus
  - Painful nodules in pouch of Douglas may indicate endometriosis
- Testicular examination for varicocoeles
- Serum progesterone levels on day 21 of menstrual cycle to assess ovulation
- TFT, prolactin
- Semen analysis may reveal low sperm count or poor motility
- Pelvic USS
- Hysterosalpingogram

MANAGEMENT

- Support and reassurance and advice on the need for regular sexual intercourse
- Manage problems with weight, smoking, alcohol and drugs
- Consider psychotherapy for those with psychosexual issues

- Clomiphene to stimulate ovulation in those with oligoovulation or anovulation such as polycystic ovarian syndrome
- In-vitro fertilisation where there is a problem with the fallopian tubes or sperm quality
- As a last resort, raise the possibility of adoption if it seems pregnancy is highly unlikely

FURTHER READING

NICE guidelines on fertility, https://www.nice.org.uk/guidance/cg156

URINARY INCONTINENCE

INITIATING THE SESSION

- Greet the patient, ask an open question and screen for other problems

MEDICAL PERSPECTIVE

SEQUENCE OF EVENTS

- **Open question** – Can you tell me more about the problem?
- **Timeline** – How did it start? How has it progressed since then?

SYMPTOM ANALYSIS

- **Onset** – How long has this been going on for?
- **Frequency** – How often do you pass water in a day? More than six times?
- **Nocturia** – How many times do you go during the night? More than twice?
- **Amount** – How much water do you pass each time? Large or small amounts?
- **Urge** – Do you ever get the strong urge to go all of a sudden? Have there been times where you haven't been able to make it in time?
- **Stress** – Have you noticed any leaks when straining, coughing or walking?
- **Pads** – Do you use pads to help keep yourself dry? How many do you use in a day? What type of pads do you use? Contipads or nappies?
- **Access** – Do you have easy access to a toilet all the time? Do you always make sure you know where the toilets are when going out?

SYSTEMS REVIEW

RED FLAGS

New onset back pain
Psychosocial dysfunction

- **Haematuria** – Have you noticed any blood in your urine?
- **Pain** – Do you get a burning pain when passing water? Have you experienced any pain in your abdomen? Do you have any new onset back pain?
- **Constipation** – Do you suffer from constipation?
- **NS** – Do you have any muscle weakness or disability?
- **Constitutional** – Do you feel ill or feverish? Any weight loss? Do you have any pains in your bones?
- **GUT (men)** – Do you find that it takes a while to get the stream going? Is the stream weak or strong? Do you have to stop and start several times when passing water? Is there prolonged dribbling at the end? Do you have the feeling that after passing water there is still some left to pass?
- **Obstetric history (women)** – *See gynaecological history template*
- **Prolapse (women)** – Do you have a heavy dragging sensation down below? Have you noticed anything protruding from there when you cough?

PATIENT'S PERSPECTIVE

- **Feelings and effect on life** – How have your symptoms affected you day-to-day? What effect has it had on your mood?
- **Ideas** – Do you have any ideas yourself about what could be causing the problem?

- **Concerns** – Is there anything you are particularly concerned could be causing it? Is there anything in general that concerns you?
- **Expectations** – Was there anything in particular you were hoping for when you made the appointment for today?

BACKGROUND INFORMATION

PMH

- Do you suffer from any medical conditions?
- *Ask about neurological disorders*

DH

- Are you currently taking any medication? Do you have any allergies?
- *Ask about diuretics ("water tablets")*

FH

- Do any conditions run in the family?
- Has anyone in your family suffered from similar problems? *If so,* what did they have done about it? Is this something you have thought about?

SH

- Do you drink much tea, coffee or fizzy drinks?
- Do you drink anything in the couple of hours before you go to bed?
- Do you drink alcohol? Smoke? How much?
- Are you currently working? *If so,* what is your job? What does that involve?
- Can you tell me about your home situation (*occupants and any difficulties*)?
- Has your problem affected your job or home life in any way?
- Are you still able to go out and meet friends or do you find yourself too restricted?

CLOSING THE SESSION

- summary ± examination/explanation and planning/contract

IMPORTANT POINTS

- This is often an embarrassing complaint for patients. Be tactful and try ways to make the patient feel comfortable talking to you. E.g. Tell the patient that one in five people suffer with incontinence and most for many years before they can talk about it
- Communication skills are very important – It often takes many years for a patient to approach a doctor about incontinence as they are so embarrassed by the problem
- The psychosocial impact of incontinence is huge – Quality of life is reduced, depression and sexual dysfunction are more common and many take time off work due to the problem
- Social history is important – Are they drinking lots of caffeine? Fluid before bed?

DIFFERENTIAL DIAGNOSIS

The aetiology of urinary incontinence is often multifactorial. Broadly speaking, it can be divided into stress incontinence, urge incontinence and mixed incontinence. Make sure this is not a presentation of spinal cord compression or cauda equina syndrome. These will present with acute back pain as well as neurological signs and symptoms and are medical emergencies.

STRESS INCONTINENCE

- Weak/damaged pelvic floor or anal sphincter
- Risk factors – Multiparity, complications of vaginal delivery, surgery, perineal tear and episiotomy
- Vaginal prolapse may be seen with symptoms of a heavy dragging sensation

URGE INCONTINENCE

- BPH or prostatic carcinoma
  - Very common in elderly males
  - Urinary symptoms include hesitancy, intermittency, weak stream, terminal dribbling and feeling of incomplete bladder emptying
  - Bone pain, weight loss, jaundice all indicate metastatic carcinoma
- Autonomic neuropathy
  - E.g. diabetes mellitus, multiple sclerosis and Parkinson's disease
  - Other neurological symptoms likely to be present
- Infection
  - Local irritation leads to urinary symptoms
  - Burning pain on micturition, fever, flank/groin/back pain, haematuria, confusion, nausea and vomiting
- Stool impaction

INVESTIGATIONS

- For women
  - Abdominal examination (palpable bladder)
  - PV examination (structural abnormalities)
  - Urine dipstick and MSU
  - Urodynamic studies
  - Urgent referral if macroscopic haematuria or microscopic haematuria >50 y/o
- For men
  - Abdominal examination
  - Digital rectal examination (enlarged prostate)
  - Bloods – FBC, LFT, U&E, bone profile (evidence of metastatic disease)
  - PSA
  - Urodynamic studies
  - Urgent transrectal USS and biopsy if hard, irregular prostate or raised age-specific PSA
  - MRI and bone scan if indicated

MANAGEMENT

- **Conservative** – Lifestyle advice (e.g. reduce caffeine intake; no fluids before bed) and pelvic floor exercises
- **Medication** – Duloxetine if surgery contraindicated and conservative measures fail
- **Surgery** – Retropubic mid-urethral tape, colposuspension and/or sling
- **BPH** – Alpha blockers (e.g. tamsulosin) and 5-alpha reductase inhibitors (e.g. finasteride); transurethral resection of the prostate if medical treatment fails
- **Prostatic carcinoma** – Watchful waiting and surveillance; radical prostatectomy; orchidectomy; hormonal therapy e.g. goserelin and/or radiotherapy

FURTHER READING

NICE guidelines on incontinence in females, https://www.nice.org.uk/Guidance/CG171

AMENORRHOEA/OLIGOMENORRHOEA

INITIATING THE SESSION

- Greet the patient, ask an open question and screen for other problems

MEDICAL PERSPECTIVE

SEQUENCE OF EVENTS AND SYMPTOM ANALYSIS

- **Open question** – Can you tell me more about the problem?
- **LMP** – When did you have your last period?
- **Cycle** – What were your periods like before? Were they regular? How often did they come? How long did they last for?
- **Menarche** – What age were you when you had your first period?

SYSTEMS REVIEW

- **Pregnancy** – Is there any chance you could be pregnant?
- **Contraception** – Do you use contraception? Which one? How long have you been taking it? What were your periods like before you started taking it?
- **Polycystic ovarian syndrome** – Are you affected by acne? Do you find you have hair growing in unusual places like your face, chest or legs? How has your weight been?
- **Thyroid dysfunction** – What has your appetite been like? Any tremor? How have your bowels been? Do you struggle with either hot or cold temperatures particularly?
- **Hypogonadotropic hypogonadism** – How often do you exercise? Have you been feeling low in mood or anxious at all recently?
- **Peri-menopause/menopause** – Have you been suffering from problems with sweating or hot flushes recently? Has anyone commented on you being more tired or irritable recently? Can I ask how your libido has been? Have you found sex painful?
- **Hyperprolactinaemia** – Have you noticed any discharge from your nipples? Have you had any problems with your vision?
- **Obstetric** – Do you have any children? Have you previously had any problems trying to conceive? *If so*, do you know why that is?

PATIENT'S PERSPECTIVE

- **Feelings and effect on life** – How have your symptoms affected your daily life?
- **Ideas** – Do you have any ideas yourself about what could be causing the problem?
- **Concerns** – Is there anything you are particularly concerned could be causing it? Is there anything in general that concerns you?
- **Expectations** – Was there anything in particular you were hoping for when you made the appointment for today?

BACKGROUND INFORMATION

PMH

- Do you suffer from any medical conditions?
- *Ask about thyroid disease, polycystic ovarian syndrome and eating disorders*

DH

- Are you currently taking any medications? Do you have any allergies?

FH

- Do any conditions run in your family?
- *Ask about autoimmune and thyroid disease?*
- Do you know what age your mum was when she reached menopause?

SH

- Are you currently working? *If so,* what is your job? What does that involve?
- Can you tell me about your home situation (*occupants and any difficulties*)?
- Has your problem affected your job or home life in any way?
- Do you smoke? How many cigarettes do you smoke a day? For how long?
- Do you drink alcohol? How much do you drink in a week?

CLOSING THE SESSION

- summary ± examination/explanation and planning/contract

> **IMPORTANT POINTS**
> - Always consider if the patient could be pregnant!
> - What contraception are they currently utilising? Could this affect their menstrual cycle?

DIFFERENTIAL DIAGNOSIS

Amenorrhoea can either be primary (menses not started by age of 16 years) or secondary (previously normal menses ceased for at least 6 months). Oligomenorrhoea is where the patient experiences menses infrequently, every 35 days to 6 months. This is common in both those who have recently undergone menarche and those who are reaching menopause but also occurs in several conditions. Depending on the age of the patient, different differentials will be more or less likely.

PRIMARY AMENORRHOEA

- Not reached menarche by age 16 years
- Most commonly constitutional delay; less commonly due to Turner's syndrome, testicular feminisation or polycystic ovarian syndrome
- In constitutional delay, the patient's mothers and sisters may also have been late in starting

PREGNANCY

- Always ask if there is any chance the patient could be pregnant and explore
- Morning sickness, abdominal distension/weight gain, possible implantation bleed 6–12 days after fertilisation, changes in mood

DRUG INDUCED

- Progesterone-only contraception in particular can cause periods to stop
- Reverses within a year upon stopping medication

POLYCYSTIC OVARIAN SYNDROME

- Symptoms due to excessive amounts of androgenic hormones
- Hirsutism, acne, weight gain, subfertility and polycystic ovaries seen on USS
- Oligomenorrhoea more commonly but can also present as amenorrhoea
- Insulin resistance and therefore obesity and diabetes associated with condition

HYPERTHYROIDISM

- Intolerance to heat, tremor, weight loss despite increased appetite, frequent bowel movements, protruding eyes, goitre and either oligomenorrhoea or amenorrhoea

HYPOTHYROIDISM

- Intolerance to cold, dry coarse skin, weight gain despite poor appetite, constipation, hair thinning, feeling slowed down and menstrual irregularities
- More often causes menorrhagia but can present as irregular periods

HYPOGONADOTROPIC HYPOGONADISM

- Low FSH and LH levels
- Most common causes – Starvation, excessive exercise, anorexia nervosa, depression, stress, chronic illness and marijuana use

MENOPAUSE

- In peri-menopausal period ("the change") symptoms are experienced
- Hot flushes, irregular periods, profuse sweating, irritability, loss of libido, vaginal atrophy
- Menopause occurs when periods have been absent for at least 12 consecutive months
- Premature menopause if onset before 40 y/o

HYPERPROLACTINAEMIA

- Galactorrhoea, amenorrhoea/oligomenorrhoea and subfertility
- Macroprolactinomas may compress optic nerve leading to bitemporal hemianopia
- Other causes – Pregnancy, breastfeeding, stress, drugs, pituitary stalk damage

INVESTIGATIONS

- Abdominal and PV examination (assess for vaginal atrophy and ovarian masses)
- Pregnancy test
- Bloods – FSH, LH, oestrogen, TFTs and prolactin
- Pelvic USS to assess for polycystic ovaries
- MRI of head to assess for pituitary and hypothalamic causes

MANAGEMENT

Other than those listed below, also consider the patient's desire for pregnancy. If they are trying to conceive then offer counselling for the couple for advice. Ovulation-inducing medications may be considered

- **Polycystic ovarian syndrome** – Weight loss and a healthy diet if obese or having difficulty conceiving; COCP can help with hirsutism and regulate periods; metformin for insulin resistance; laparoscopic ovarian drilling
- **Hyperthyroidism** – Propranolol and carbimazole initially; radioiodine or surgery where medical treatment fails
- **Hypothyroidism** – Thyroxine
- **Hypogonadotropic hypogonadism** – Lifestyle advice and CBT if indicated
- **Menopause** – Topical lubricant, cream or oestrogen for vaginal atrophy and/or systemic hormone replacement therapy
- **Hyperprolactinaemia** – Bromocriptine and surgery if visual defect present

FURTHER READING

NICE CKS on amenorrhoea, http://cks.nice.org.uk/amenorrhoea

Paediatrics

11

PAEDIATRIC HISTORY TEMPLATE

For the general paediatric history, the following components should be considered as part of the review. These are referred to in the subsequent histories in this section.

TRAFFIC LIGHT SYSTEM

- **Colour** – Does the child look more pale to the parent/carer?
- **Activity** – Are they playing and interacting as normal or more tired than usual?
- **Respiratory** – Has the parent/carer noticed any difficulty with their breathing?
- **Hydration/circulation** – How are they feeding? Are they drinking as much as usual? Are they having as many wet nappies as normal for them?
- **Other** – Have they felt hot? Have they had any recorded temperatures? Any rashes?

PREGNANCY AND BIRTH HISTORY

- **Prenatal**
  - Any maternal illnesses during pregnancy? (*diabetes, pre-eclampsia, infections*)
  - Did the mother smoke, take alcohol or drugs during pregnancy?
  - Complications during pregnancy and labour
- **Natal**
  - Was it a normal delivery, assisted or caesarean section?
  - Did the pregnancy reach term? What was his/her birth weight?
- **Postnatal**
  - Was the child well?
  - Did he/she require admission?

FEEDING HISTORY (INFANTS AND TODDLERS)

- **Bottle/breast** – Is/was the child bottle-fed or breastfed? *Details of feeding*
- **Weaning** – At what age were solids introduced? Was there any difficulty weaning?
- **Feeding pattern** – What does he/she eat? Any trouble with certain foods e.g. dairy?

DEVELOPMENT HISTORY

- **Concerns** – Has anyone had any concerns about his/her development?
- **Milestones** – Has he/she met all his/her developmental milestones so far? *Take a full developmental history if appropriate, otherwise just check a couple of milestones across the different categories (gross motor; vision and fine motor; social, emotional and behavioural; hearing, speech and language) e.g. when did he/she say his/her first word? When did he/she start walking unsupported?*

IMMUNISATION HISTORY

- Is the child up to date with all his/her vaccinations?
- When was his/her last one? What was it for?

IMPORTANT POINTS

- Always establish first who it is you are talking to – Is it the mother, father, relative, social worker, foster parent or the child?
- Make sure you know the age of the child as this will shape the rest of the history
- Adapt the history for the child's age and situation e.g. if they are an adolescent with a cough, a full developmental and feeding history would be inappropriate
- In the family history, try to look for any possible pattern of inheritance and consider drawing a family tree if given relevant
- Consider whether there is any consanguinity
- Take a detailed social history including the home, school and social environments

FURTHER READING

NICE CKS on feverish children, http://cks.nice.org.uk/feverish-children-risk-assessment

VOMITING

INITIATING THE SESSION

- Greet the patient, ask an open question and screen for other problems

MEDICAL PERSPECTIVE

SEQUENCE OF EVENTS

- **Open question** – Can you tell me more about his/her vomiting?
- **Timeline** – When did he/she start vomiting? How has it progressed since then?

SYMPTOM ANALYSIS

- **Appearance** – What colour is the vomitus? (*blood, bile, milky*)
- **Projection** – Does it hit the wall? (*projectile/regurgitation/posseting*)
- **Timing** – Is there any particular time when the vomiting starts? Any relation to feeds? How does he/she feel afterwards? Is he/she hungry for more food?
- **Exacerbating factors** – Does anything bring the vomiting on? Is it worse when the child is lying down or sitting up? Does anything help?

SYSTEMS REVIEW (*SEE PAEDIATRIC HISTORY TEMPLATE*)

- **GIT** – What are his/her stools like? Does he/she complain of tummy ache?
- **Urine** – Have you noticed any strange/offensive smell in his/her urine? Has he/she complained of any pain?
- **Scales** – Is he/she growing normally? Has he/she been gaining weight?
- **Traffic light system**
- **Feeding history** (*infants and toddlers*)
- **Pregnancy and birth history**
- **Development history**
- **Immunisation history**

> **RED FLAGS**
>
> *Projectile vomiting*
> *Less than 50% feeds taken*
> *Absence of wet nappies*
> *Red features on traffic light*
> *Non-blanching rash*
> *Symptoms of UTI*

PATIENT'S PERSPECTIVE

- **Feelings and effect on life** – What effect has this had on him/her at school? At home?
- **Ideas** – Do you have any ideas yourself about what could be causing the vomits?
- **Concerns** – Is there anything you are particularly concerned could be causing it? Is there anything in general that concerns you?
- **Expectations** – Was there anything in particular you were hoping for when you made the appointment for today?

BACKGROUND INFORMATION

PMH

- How has he/she been before this episode? Any previous illnesses?

DH

- Has he/she been given any medications? Does he/she have any allergies?

FH

- Do any conditions run in the family?
- *Ask about coeliac disease and IBD if relevant*

SH

- Who is at home? Are you still with his/her mother/father? Does he/she have any siblings? How are things at home?
- Is the child at school, playgroup or nursery? How are things there?
- Has anyone at home or at school had similar symptoms?

CLOSING THE SESSION

- summary ± examination/explanation and planning/contract

IMPORTANT POINTS

- The age of the child is very important in this case, as some conditions are more common in certain age groups
- It is always important to check the relationship between the adult and child and to make sure that the adult you are speaking to is the legal guardian or has parental responsibility of the child
- Remember to quantify the feeds; vomiting may simply be due to overfeeding of the child
- Always remember to rule out more serious conditions such as meningitis

---

DIFFERENTIAL DIAGNOSIS

GASTRO-OESOPHAGEAL REFLUX DISEASE

- Very common in first year of life due to functional immaturity of lower oesophageal sphincter
- Recurrent regurgitation and vomiting related to feeds; relieved by sitting up
- Child can be distressed after feeding – feeding and behavioural difficulties
- Other risk factors include premature delivery and cerebral palsy

PYLORIC STENOSIS

- Peak age 2–7 weeks
- Projectile vomiting straight after feed
- Child remains hungry after vomiting
- Complications: dehydration, constipation and failure to thrive

INTUSSUSCEPTION

- Peak age 5–10 months
- Paroxysms of colicky abdominal pain around every 10–20 minutes; often indicated by child drawing knees into their chest and inconsolable crying
- Early – Vomiting which rapidly becomes bile stained
- Later – Mucus and blood per rectum (redcurrant jelly stools)

COELIAC DISEASE

- Peak age 9 months–3 years (typically after weaning)
- Vomiting, pallor, steatorrhoea, abdominal distension and failure to thrive

MENINGITIS

- Vomiting – Will not take feeds
- Fever, irritable or lethargic
- Non-blanching purpuric rash
- Cold extremities
- Signs of increased intracranial pressure i.e. bulging fontanelle

GASTROENTERITIS

- Diarrhoea and vomiting
- Fever, irritable and unwell
- History of recent travel
- There may well be someone in family or school with similar symptoms

INVESTIGATIONS

- Physical examination of child – If satisfied from history and examination it is GORD or uncomplicated gastroenteritis no further investigations are required
- U&Es (to look for any signs of dehydration)
- Pyloric stenosis – Test feed, feeling for olive-shaped mass in epigastrium and looking for visible peristalsis; USS to confirm
- Intussusception – USS abdomen and barium enema
- Coeliac disease – Tissue transglutaminase autoantibodies; duodenal biopsy to confirm
- Meningitis – Neuro exam and look for rash, lumbar puncture (CT head first if possible raised intracranial pressure), blood cultures and blood glucose

MANAGEMENT

- **Rehydration** – With oral intake if mild–moderate; IV fluids if severe
  - Rehydration is usually all that is required in GORD and gastroenteritis
- **Pyloric stenosis** – Pyloromyotomy
- **Intussusception** – Air enema/barium enema if diagnosed early, otherwise surgery

- **Coeliac disease** – Lifelong gluten-free diet
- **Meningitis** – Antibiotics (e.g. benzylpenicillin IM initially and cefotaxime IV) in bacterial meningitis; antipyretics and analgesia in viral meningitis

FURTHER READING

NICE guidance on:
Pathways for diarrhoea and vomiting in children, http://pathways.nice.org.uk/pathways/diarrhoea-and-vomiting-in-children
Reflux in babies, https://www.nice.org.uk/guidance/ng1/ifp/chapter/reflux-in-babies
Gastroenteritis (children), https://www.nice.org.uk/guidance/cg84/chapter/1-guidance

FAILURE TO THRIVE

"My child isn't growing/putting on weight like other kids his/her age."

INITIATING THE SESSION

- Greet the patient, ask an open question and screen for other problems

MEDICAL PERSPECTIVE

SEQUENCE OF EVENTS AND SYMPTOM ANALYSIS

- **Open question** – Can you tell me more about your concerns?
- **Clarify** – Are you concerned about his/her height, weight or both?
- **Timeline** – When did you first notice this? How has it progressed since then? Has he/she always been a small child? What was his/her birth weight? How has his/her growth been since birth? Has he/she been putting any weight/height on? Has he/she lost any weight?

SYSTEMS REVIEW (*SEE PAEDIATRIC HISTORY TEMPLATE*)

- **GIT** – Can I ask what his/her stools look like? Has he/she had any diarrhoea? Has he/she been vomiting at all? Any tummy ache?
- **RS** – Has he/she had a cough? *If so*, for how long? Does he/she bring anything up?
- **Constitutional** – Has he/she had any recurrent infections?
- **Traffic light system**
- **Feeding history**
- **Pregnancy and birth history**
- **Development history**
- **Immunisation history**

PATIENT'S PERSPECTIVE

- **Feelings and effect on life** – How has he/she been at home? At school?
- **Ideas** – Do you have any ideas yourself about what could be causing the difficulty gaining weight?
- **Concerns** – Is there anything you are particularly concerned could be causing it? Is there anything in general that concerns you?
- **Expectations** – Other than trying to get to the bottom of why he/she isn't putting on weight as quickly as we'd like, is there anything else you were hoping for when you made the appointment for today?

BACKGROUND INFORMATION

PMH

- Does he/she have any medical or genetic problems you know of?

DH

- Has he/she been given any medications? Does he/she have any allergies?

FH

- Do any conditions run in the family?
- *Ask specifically about coeliac disease, cystic fibrosis and diabetes*
- How were you and your partner growing up? Did you have any problems?

SH

- Who is at home? Does he/she have any siblings? How are they?
- How are things at home? Do you feel you have enough support?
- Is he/she at school, playgroup or nursery? How is he/she doing there?

CLOSING THE SESSION

- summary ± examination/explanation and planning/contract

IMPORTANT POINTS

- The age of the child is very important in this case as feeding patterns, amount and products differ at different ages
- The history of the pregnancy is important here – did they smoke, drink alcohol or have any illnesses?
- It is always important to check the relationship between the adult and child and to make sure that the adult you are speaking to is the legal guardian or has parental responsibility of the child
- Note how the parent speaks about the child – Are they caring and concerned or cold and distant? This could help to determine whether the child is at risk
- Substitute "your child" with the child's actual name

DIFFERENTIAL DIAGNOSIS

ORGANIC CAUSES

Prenatal

- Prematurity, maternal malnutrition, congenital infections, intrauterine growth restriction and toxin exposure in-utero [e.g. alcohol (foetal alcoholic syndrome), cigarettes or recreational drugs]

Intake issues

- Inability to suck or swallow in neuromuscular disorders (e.g. cerebral palsy)
- Cleft palate, long-standing GORD or vomiting after feeds

Malabsorption

- Diarrhoea will be a prominent feature – Note when this occurs
- Cystic fibrosis – Cough with sputum, URTI
- Coeliac disease (typically as solids are introduced); IBD, cow's milk intolerance and unspecified chronic diarrhoea can also cause malabsorption

Metabolic disorders

- Poor metabolism in hypothyroidism and diabetes
- Increased metabolic demand in hyperthyroidism, heart and renal failure

NON-ORGANIC CAUSES

Constitutional delay

- Genetic predisposition (i.e. short parents, short child!)
- No other problems identified in history

Inadequate feeds

- Not being fed enough or often enough
- Distractions at meal time
- Poor breastfeeding technique
- Bottle feeds not made up correctly
- Could be due to lack of knowledge/supervision or child neglect
- Contributing factors include lack of support and problems in home environment

INVESTIGATIONS

- Physical examination, including cardiac (murmurs), respiratory (wheeze, crepitations), abdominal (masses) and neurological (cranial nerves and limbs)
- Plot measurements on growth and weight centile charts
- Observe the child feeding if possible in infant feeding
- If an obvious cause is identified no further tests may be required
- Blood tests – FBC, U&Es, ESR, TFTs, LFTs, glucose
- Urinalysis and urine culture
- Stool culture for ova/parasites/cysts and faecal fat for malabsorption
- Anti-gliadin and anti-endomysial autoantibodies for coeliac disease
- Sweat test for cystic fibrosis

MANAGEMENT

- General measures
  - Provide a suitable feeding environment
  - Parent education on feeding requirements, breastfeeding technique etc.
- A multidisciplinary approach may be required
  - Health visitors may help if the parents are not coping well at home
  - Dieticians provide invaluable input – particularly in celiac disease
  - Paediatricians for assessment and management of organic conditions
  - Where child neglect is suspected, social services should be involved

FURTHER READING

NICE guidance on faltering growth, to be released in October 2017, https://www.nice.org.uk/guidance/indevelopment/gid-cgwave0767

Patient.co.uk profession article on faltering growth in children, http://patient.info/doctor/faltering-growth-in-children

CONVULSIONS

INITIATING THE SESSION

- Greet the patient, ask an open question and screen for other problems

MEDICAL PERSPECTIVE

SEQUENCE OF EVENTS

- **Open question** – Can you tell me more about the episode?
- **Timeline** – When did it first happen? Has he/she had any further episodes?

SYMPTOM ANALYSIS

Before

- **Witness** – Did you witness the episode? Can you talk me through what happened?
- **Precipitating factors** – What was he/she doing before it started? Was he/she scared or crying? Had he/she fallen or hit his/her head before the episode? Had he/she been unwell?
- **Aura** – Did he/she describe any funny feelings or sensations before the episode?

During

- **Duration** – How long did the episode last for?
- **LOC** – Did he/she lose consciousness? Did he/she fall to the floor? *If so*, did he/she hit his/her head?
- **Seizures** – Was he/she shaking? *If so*, can you describe it please? Did his/her whole body jerk or only part of it?
- **Tongue biting** – Did he/she bite his/her tongue? *If so*, the front or the side of his/her tongue?
- **Incontinence** – Did he/she pass water or soil himself?
- **Pallor/cyanosis** – Did he/she appear pale or blue during the episode?

After

- **Postictal state** – How did he/she feel immediately after the episode? Does he/she remember the event?
- **Previous episodes** – Has this ever happened before?
- **General health** – How is he/she doing generally? Is he/she growing and gaining weight normally? Is he/she sleeping well?

SYSTEMS REVIEW (*SEE PAEDIATRIC HISTORY TEMPLATE*)

- **Traffic light system**
- **Pregnancy and birth history**
- **Development history**
- **Immunisation history**
- **Feeding history** (*infants and toddlers*)

RED FLAGS

Red features on traffic light
Seizure lasting >15 minutes
Focal seizure
Recurrent within same illness
Otorrhoea
Suspected meningitis

PATIENT'S PERSPECTIVE

- **Feelings and effect on life** – How has he/she been at home? At school?
- **Ideas** – Do you have any ideas yourself about what could be causing the episode(s)?
- **Concerns** – Is there anything you are particularly concerned could be causing them? Is there anything in general that concerns you?
- **Expectations** – Other than trying to get to the bottom of why this happened, is there anything else you were hoping for when you made the appointment for today?

BACKGROUND INFORMATION

PMH

- Does he/she have any other medical problems?
- *Ask specifically about cerebral palsy, tuberous sclerosis and previous meningitis*

DH

- Is he/she on any medication at the moment? Does he/she have any allergies?

FH

- Do any conditions run in the family?
- *Ask specifically about a family history of epilepsy and febrile convulsions*

SH

- Who is at home? Are there any problems at home? Does he/she have any siblings?
- Is he/she at school, playgroup or nursery? How are things there?

CLOSING THE SESSION

- summary ± examination/explanation and planning/contract

IMPORTANT POINTS

- It is always important to check the relationship between the adult and child and to make sure that the adult you are speaking to is the legal guardian or has parental responsibility of the child
- The pregnancy and birth history is very important here as any injuries or toxins during this time could have predisposed the child to having convulsions
- The parent is likely to be very distressed and concerned in this history, as it is distressing for anyone to witness their child convulsing – an empathetic and understanding nature is imperative
- Commonly the parent's primary concern is that their child has epilepsy – often it is the child's first seizure and there is a clear history of fever, so it is acceptable to explain that he/she is likely suffering from febrile convulsions (explain what this means and measures the parents can take to prevent re-occurrences) and that a diagnosis of epilepsy cannot be made on the basis of one seizure alone in any case

DIFFERENTIAL DIAGNOSIS

FEBRILE CONVULSIONS

- Affects children between the ages of 6 months to 5 years
- High temperature (>38°C) at time of seizure, usually due to a common viral infection
- Tonic and/or clonic, symmetrical, generalised seizure usually lasting <5 minutes
- No signs of central nervous system infection, focal neurological signs or a previous history of epilepsy (a discharging ear should prompt urgent imaging and should not automatically give rise to a diagnosis of febrile convulsion)

REFLEX ANOXIC SEIZURE

- Brief and spontaneous, paroxysmal episodes triggered by fear, anxiety or pain
- Episode lasts <1 minute
- Typically, the child suddenly becomes pale and limp, losing consciousness briefly
- This is then followed by involuntary tonic and/or clonic movements of the limbs
- Urinary incontinence may be evident and the child may feel groggy afterwards
- Unlike in epilepsy, tongue biting is not a feature

BREATH HOLDING ATTACK

- Often precipitated by emotions such as anger or frustration or trauma
- A crying episode often ensues, breath is withheld and pallor or cyanosis develops
- Loss of consciousness may occur, but recovery is usually quick

EPILEPSY

- Risk factors include birth asphyxia, cerebral palsy and trauma
- Watching television and lack of sleep are known precipitants
- Partial seizures cause symptoms depending on the part of the cerebrum affected e.g. strange sensations, deja vu, paraesthesia down one limb; lasts up to a few minutes
  - Simple – No loss of consciousness
  - Complex – Impaired level of consciousness
- Generalised seizures involve the entire cerebrum
  - Absence – Frequent episodes where the child stops what he/she is doing, remains still and stares vacantly for 2–3 seconds
  - Tonic-clonic – Classic episodes of stiffening of the body lasting for 10–20 seconds, followed by violent shaking of limbs; tongue biting, incontinence and post-ictal state are associated with this type; can last up to 2–3 minutes
- There are many other variants associated with childhood epilepsy

MENINGITIS

- Unwell and drowsy child prior to convulsions with pyrexia
- Non-blanching rash of meningococcal septicaemia may be present
- If the patient has a discharging ear, consider whether they could have intracranial complications of otitis media

OTHERS

- Tuberous sclerosis – Condition which causes multiple non-cancerous tumours to develop around the body including the brain
- Vasovagal syncope
- Benign paroxysmal vertigo
- Hypoglycaemic attack

INVESTIGATIONS

- Neurological examination (including Kernig's sign, Brudzinski's sign and looking for bulging fontanelle) and inspection for any rashes
- If normal examination, including observations, and typical history of febrile convulsions, no further investigations may be required
- Lumbar puncture and blood cultures if there is any suspicion of meningitis
- Blood tests – FBC, U&Es, LFTs, glucose (hypoglycaemia)
- ECG to rule out underlying arrhythmias
- EEG – Best done during a seizure

MANAGEMENT

- Hospital admission and paediatric assessment is warranted if this is the first convulsion even if thought to be due to febrile seizures
- Parent education
- Put the child in the recovery position when convulsing and call for help
- Keep temperature down when pyrexial and give plenty of fluids and paracetamol
- Usually for reflex anoxic seizures and breath holding attacks, parental reassurance is all that is required
- Epilepsy
  - Not everyone requires treatment
  - Specialist paediatric or neurological referral is required
  - Generally, sodium valproate is reserved for those with partial seizures and carbamazepine for those with generalised seizures

FURTHER READING

NICE CKS on febrile seizures, http://cks.nice.org.uk/febrile-seizure

DEVELOPMENTAL DELAY E.G. DELAYED WALKING

INITIATING THE SESSION

- Greet the patient, ask an open question and screen for other problems

MEDICAL PERSPECTIVE

SEQUENCE OF EVENTS

- **Open question** – Can you tell me more about your concerns?
- **Timeline** – Can you talk me through how he/she has developed since birth and when he/she reached any milestones you noticed? How old is your child now? (*Consider now whether the child is truly late in meeting the milestone*)

SYMPTOM ANALYSIS

- **Development** – How has your child been developing otherwise? Tell me about him/her. What can he/she manage to do now? Do you have his/her red book with you?
- **Concerns** – Are you concerned about his/her development in any other areas?
- **Family pattern** – Do you know what age *his/her parents* first started walking? Siblings?
- I would like to ask some quick questions to check your child's development, is that OK? *See below. NB: only ask those relevant to the child's age*

GROSS MOTOR

- Have you got any concerns with his/her physical development?
- **Hand dominance** – Does he/she favour either hand? How long has he/she been like that for?
- **Early motor** – What age did your child first hold his/her head up? Sit up? Crawl? How does he/she crawl? *On both knees? With one leg trailing behind? Bottom-shuffling?*
- **Walk** – When did he/she start to walk unsupported?

VISION AND FINE MOTOR

- Have you got any concerns with his/her eyesight or development of finer skills?
- **Fix and follow** – When did you notice he/she first started following things with his/her eyes?
- **Objects** – When did he/she start reaching for things? Transferring things from one hand to the other? Make a pincer grip?
- **Drawings** – What does he/she draw when given a pencil and paper? Is he/she able to scribble a line or a circle? Can he/she copy a line or circle if you draw it?
- **Stacking toys** – Can be build towers with his/her blocks? How many levels can he/she build?

HEARING, SPEECH AND LANGUAGE

- **Hearing** – Have you got any concerns with his/her hearing? Does he/she react to sounds out of sight? Does he/she respond when you call him/her?
- **Speech** – What can he/she say now? What age did he/she first babble? When did he/she say his/her first word?

SOCIAL, EMOTIONAL AND BEHAVIOURAL

- Can you describe his/her social interactions with others?
- **Actions** – What age did you first see him/her smile? Wave bye-bye?
- **Play** – Does he/she pretend to play with teddy? Does he/she play and share with others?

SYSTEMS REVIEW (*SEE PAEDIATRIC HISTORY TEMPLATE*)

- **Traffic light system**
- **Pregnancy and birth history**
- **Immunisation history**
- **Feeding history** (*infants and toddlers*)

PATIENT'S PERSPECTIVE

- **Feelings and effect on life** – How has he/she been at home? At school?
- **Ideas** – Do you have any ideas yourself about what could be going on?
- **Concerns** – Is there anything you are particularly concerned about? Is there anything in general that concerns you?
- **Expectations** – Can I check if there was anything in particular you were hoping for today?

BACKGROUND INFORMATION

PMH

- Has he/she had any serious illnesses?
- *Ask specifically about meningitis*

DH

- Is he/she taking any medications? Any allergies?

FH

- Do any conditions run in the family?
- *Ask specifically about Duchenne's muscular atrophy*
- When did Mum and Dad start walking?

SH

- Who is at home? How are things at home?
- Does he/she get the chance to move around?
- Is he/she at pre-school, nursery or a playgroup? How is he/she doing there?

CLOSING THE SESSION

- summary ± examination/explanation and planning/contract

RED FLAGS

Red light features
Loss of skill at any age
Not fixing or following objects
Can't sit unsupported by 12 months
No speech by 18 months
Not standing by 18 months
Persistent toe walking
Loss of hearing

Developmental milestones at ages usually achieved by, with important/more reliable milestones listed in bold (below)

Age (months)	Gross motor	Vision and fine motor	Hearing, speech and language	Social, emotional and behavioural
1.5	Head level with body in ventral suspension	**Fixes eyes and follows visually**	Gurgles	**Smiles**
3	Holds head up at 90° in ventral suspension	Holds objects placed in hand	**Turns to sounds;** coos	Laughs and squeals
6	**Good head control** (No head lag on pull-to-sit)	Transfer objects hand-to-hand	Vocalises	Enjoys eye contact and facial expressions
9	**Sits unsupported**	Early pincer grip	Babbles e.g. mama	Waves bye-bye
12	Stands independently	**Effective pincer grip**	**Imitates sounds,** may develop 1 or 2 words	**Plays peekaboo**
18	**Walks unsupported**	**Stacks tower of 2–3 cubes; scribbles line; uses spoon**	>5 words spoken	Mimics actions of others e.g. wiping
24	Walks, jumps, kicks, throws	Stacks tower of 6 cubes; scribbles circle	50 words; **2-word phrases**	**Symbolic play**
36	Pedals tricycle	Stacks tower of 10 cubes; copies circles; uses fork and spoon	Talks in intelligible short sentences	Peer interactions and role play

DIFFERENTIAL DIAGNOSIS

The differential for developmental delay is very large, depending on which of the four fields of development are affected. If all four fields are affected, it implies a global developmental delay. If one field is affected significantly more than the others, there is a specific developmental delay. Differential diagnosis for two of the commonest presentations of developmental delay is considered below:

DELAY IN MOTOR DEVELOPMENT

NORMAL VARIATION

- Often a family history of delayed development of motor skills
- Normal in all other aspects but slow in developing motor skills
- When motor skills are achieved, they are of a normal standard
- Children who are bottom-shufflers or commando-crawlers are more likely to develop walking skills later than children who crawl on their knees and hands

CEREBRAL PALSY

- Disorder of motor function caused by non-progressive pathology to the developing brain
- Abnormal tone and posture and delayed achievement of motor milestones
- Often widespread dysfunction e.g. learning difficulties and epilepsy
- Three types: spastic, ataxic hypotonic and dyskinetic cerebral palsy
- Causes (usually in antenatal period):
  - Antenatal – vascular occlusion, congenital infection, maldevelopment of the brain
  - Perinatal – prolonged hypoxia in birth
  - Postnatal – head trauma, meningoencephalitis, periventricular leucomalacia
- Premature babies are at an increased risk of developing periventricular leucomalacia

DUCHENNE MUSCULAR DYSTROPHY

- X-linked recessive condition (affects boys only)
- Delayed achievement of motor milestones, waddling gait and possible global delay
- Gower's sign: child uses hands to "climb up" legs in order to stand up

OTHER

- Causes of global developmental delay – e.g. Down's syndrome, tuberous sclerosis
- Metabolic disorder – e.g. rickets, hypoglycaemia
- Environmental – e.g. a child who is always kept in the cot or bedbound through illness

DELAY IN SPEECH AND LANGUAGE DEVELOPMENT

NORMAL VARIATION

- Often a family history of delayed speech development
- Otherwise normal and appropriately developing child

HEARING DIFFICULTIES

- Otitis media with effusion is common in childhood and can cause delayed speech and language development and later affect performance in school

AUTISTIC SPECTRUM DISORDER

- Impaired reciprocal social interaction and communication and repetitive stereotyped behaviours
- Delayed or complete lack of speech development with no other forms of communication such as miming or gesturing attempted in its place
- Abnormal social, emotional and behavioural development – e.g. playing in isolation

OTHER

- Cleft palate
- Learning difficulties
- Environmental deprivation and neglect

INVESTIGATIONS

- Observation of child at play
- Neurological examination
- Ear examination and hearing assessment for speech and language delay
- Creatinine phosphokinase levels (Duchenne muscular dystrophy)
- Chromosomal karyotyping

MANAGEMENT

- MDT approach including physiotherapists, paediatricians, audiologists, psychologists, social workers, speech and language therapists and occupational therapists
- Treat underlying condition where possible (e.g. otitis media, rickets, hypoglycaemia)

FURTHER READING

Patient.co.uk professional article on delay in walking, http://patient.info/doctor/delay-in-walking

Patient.co.uk professional article on delay in talking, http://patient.info/doctor/delay-in-talking

PYREXIA (PAEDIATRIC)

INITIATING THE SESSION

- Greet the patient, ask an open question and screen for other problems

MEDICAL PERSPECTIVE

SEQUENCE OF EVENTS AND SYMPTOM ANALYSIS

- **Open question** – Can you tell me more about the fever?
- **Clarify** – What exactly do you mean when you say "fever"?
- **Timeline** – When did he/she first become unwell? What did you notice at the time? How have things progressed since then?
- **Other symptoms** – How is your child feeling generally? Any vomiting? Pain? Any night sweats? *Clarify dates*

SYSTEMS REVIEW (*SEE PAEDIATRIC HISTORY TEMPLATE*)

- **Haematological** – Have you noticed any bruising or bleeding? Is he/she getting recurrent infections? Has he/she been more tired than normal?
- **RS/CVS** – Has he/she had a cough? Can you describe it? Have you noticed any wheeze or other strange sounds with his/her breathing? Any sputum? Any chest pain?
- **ENT** – Has he/she had a runny nose? Sore throat? Earache? Any discharge from the ears? Any change in his/her hearing?
- **GIT** – Has he/she had any tummy ache? Diarrhoea or vomiting?
- **GUT** – Has he/she been complaining of any burning pains when passing urine?
- **NS** – Does he/she have a headache? Neck stiffness? A rash?
- **Constitutional** – Has he/she been anywhere abroad recently? Any insect bites? Is he/she growing well? Has he/she lost any weight?
- **Traffic light system**
- **Pregnancy and birth history**
- **Development history**
- **Immunisation history**
- **Feeding history** (*infants and toddlers*)

> **RED FLAGS**
> *Red light features*
> *Neck stiffness/*
> *photophobia*
> *Non-blanching rash*
> *Foreign travel*
> *Drenching night sweats*
> *Bleeding/bruising*
> *tendency*

PATIENT'S PERSPECTIVE

- **Feelings and effect on life** – How has he/she been at home? At school?
- **Ideas** – Do you have any ideas yourself about what could be causing the fever?
- **Concerns** – Is there anything you are particularly concerned could be causing it? Is there anything in general that concerns you?
- **Expectations** – Other than coming to a specific diagnosis, was there anything else you were hoping for when you made the appointment for today?

BACKGROUND INFORMATION

PMH

- How has he/she been before this episode? Any ongoing medical problems?
- *Ask about previous infections*

DH

- Does he/she take any medications or inhalers? Does he/she have any allergies?

FH

- Do any conditions run in the family?

SH

- Who is at home? Any pets? *If so,* how long have you had the pet?
- Does anyone smoke at home?
- Is he/she at school, playgroup or nursery?
- Does anyone in the family or at school have similar symptoms?

CLOSING THE SESSION

- summary ± examination/explanation and planning/contract

IMPORTANT POINTS

- It is always important to check the relationship between the adult and child and to make sure that the adult you are speaking to is the legal guardian or has parental responsibility of the child
- The description of the cough is very important as it could distinguish what the diagnosis is from quite early on
- Finding out whether there are any pets at home or any allergies that the child has is also very useful

DIFFERENTIAL DIAGNOSIS

URTI

- General coryzal symptoms – rhinorrhoea, dry cough, headache, sore throat
- May develop earache and otitis media secondary to this (especially if <6 y/o)

MENINGITIS

- Unwell child, irritable, drowsy, headache, photophobia, weak/high-pitched cry
- Non-blanching rash and seizures
- Can present differently, particularly early on, with abdominal pain or other non-specific symptoms that don't fit with a diagnosis (high index of suspicion important)

UTI

- Abdominal pain
- May have dysuria and strong-smelling urine
- Irritability and poor feeding

BRONCHIOLITIS

- Common viral illness seen in the first year of life
- Raspy cough, wheeze, coryzal symptoms and fever
- Less wet nappies, poor feeding and grunting sounds indicate severe infection

CROUP

- Viral illness causing a barking cough with stridor and coryzal symptoms
- Commonest in first few years of life and usually self-limiting, worse at night-time
- Can cause airway obstruction however, which must be taken seriously

KAWASAKI'S DISEASE

- Fever >5 days and four of the following five features:
- Injected pharynx/cracked lips/strawberry tongue; conjunctival injection; change in extremities; polymorphous rash; cervical lymphadenopathy

OTHERS

- Tonsillitis – sore throat and fever
- Otitis media – otalgia (or infant pulling on their ear), decreased hearing
- Pneumonia – productive cough, fever, unwell with grunting sounds
- Epiglottitis – drooling, unwell, soft stridor, severe sore throat, not had Hib vaccination
- Septic arthritis/osteomyelitis – limb/joint swelling; not using extremity/weight bearing

INVESTIGATIONS

- Physical examination (ENT, CVS, RS, abdominal and neurological examination)
- No investigations usually necessary to diagnose bronchiolitis or croup
- Chest x-ray if pneumonia likely and unwell
- Urine microscopy and MSU if no obvious source found/UTI suspected
- CT head and lumbar puncture if meningitis suspected

MANAGEMENT

- Most URTIs are self-limiting, therefore give parental advice – monitor their temperature, give paracetamol if needed and plenty of fluids
- Urgent admission for IV cephalosporins for suspected meningitis (give dose of benzylpenicillin if in community before admission)
- Bronchiolitis – may require admission for supportive management
- Croup – single dose of dexamethasone; admit if respiratory distress
- Antibiotics for UTIs and pneumonia
- Otitis media and tonsillitis – usually self-limiting, but antibiotics are required in some circumstances (*see earache and sore throat histories, pp. 129 and 137, respectively*)
- Epiglottitis and septic arthritis require urgent admission for IV antibiotics

FURTHER READING

NICE guidelines on feverish children under 5 y/o, https://www.nice.org.uk/guidance/cg160

Traffic light system for identifying of serious illness in children[a]			
	Green – low risk	**Amber – intermediate risk**	**Red – high risk**
Colour (of skin, lips or tongue)	• Normal colour	• Pallor reported by parent/carer	• Pale/mottled/ashen/blue
Activity	• Responds normally to social cues • Content/smiles • Stays awake or awakens quickly • Strong normal cry/not crying	• Not responding normally to social cues • No smile • Wakes only with prolonged stimulation • Decreased activity	• No response to social cues • Does not wake or if roused does not stay awake • Appears ill to a healthcare professional • Week, high-pitched or continuous cry

Respiratory		• Nasal flaring
		• Tachypnoea:
		  – RR >50 breaths/minute, age 6–12 months
		  – RR >40 breaths/minute, age >12 months
		• Oxygen saturation ≤95% in air
		• Crackles in the chest
			• Grunting
			• Tachypnoea: RR >60 breaths/minute
			• Moderate or severe chest indrawing

Circulation and hydration	• Normal skin and eyes
	• Moist mucous membranes
		• Tachypnoea:
		  – >160 beats/minute, age <12 months
		  – >150 beats/minute, age 12–24 months
		  – >140 beats/minute, age 2–5 months
		• CRT ≥3 seconds
		• Dry mucous membranes poor feeding in infants Reduced urine output
			• Reduced skin turgor

Other	• None of the amber or red symptoms or signs	• Age 3–6 months, temperature ~39°C • Fever for ~5 days • Rigors • Swelling of a limb or joint • Non-weight bearing limb/not using an extremity	• Age <3 months, temperature ≥38°C • Non-blanching rash • Bulging fontanelle • Neck stiffness • Status epilepticus • Focus neurological signs • Focus seizures

Note: CRT, capillary refill time; RR, respiratory rate.

[a] *This traffic light table should be used in conjunction with the recommendations in the guideline on investigations and initial management in children with fever.*

BEHAVIOUR

"I'm finding it hard to cope with my child's behaviour, he/she never listens to me."
"The school has complained about my child's behaviour."

INITIATING THE SESSION

- Greet the patient, ask an open question and screen for other problems

MEDICAL PERSPECTIVE

SEQUENCE OF EVENTS AND SYMPTOM ANALYSIS

- Tell me about what has happened regarding your child?
- When was a problem first noticed? By whom? Where? Looking back, has he/she always been this way? Have things changed over time?
- How would you describe his/her behaviour now?
- Can you think of anything that may have triggered this behaviour?

ENVIRONMENTS

- Is he/she the same way at school and home?
- **Home** – How is he/she at home? Who else is at home? What are his/her relationships like with them?
- **School** – How is he/she at school? Is it a mainstream school? What do the teachers say about him/her? How is he/she doing academically?
- **Social** – How is he/she elsewhere? Can you take him/her out to public places like restaurants?

CONDUCT

- Does he/she get into trouble often? *If so,* in what ways exactly?
- *If conduct is an issue, explore in more detail:*
  - **Disobedience** – Does he/she respect any rules or authority?
  - **Truancy** – Has he/she ever missed school?
  - **Bullying** – Does he/she get involved in bullying?
  - **Violence** – Can he/she be violent or cruel to either humans or animals?
  - **Law** – Has he/she ever been in trouble with the law? *If so,* what for?
  - **Substances** – Has he/she ever drunk alcohol, smoked or used illicit drugs?

ATTENTION DEFICIT HYPERACTIVITY DISORDER FEATURES

- **Hyperactivity** – Would you say he/she is hyperactive? Is he/she restless, fidgety and constantly talking? Is he/she constantly "bouncing off the walls"?
- **Impulsiveness** – Does he/she take turns or constantly interrupt conversations?
- **Inattention** – How are his/her concentration levels? Is he/she easily distracted?

AUTISTIC FEATURES

- **Communication** – Does he/she have any difficulties with communication?
- **Social impairment** – Does he/she have friends? Is he/she able to play with other children? Does he/she enjoy imaginary play?
- **Repetitive behaviours** – Does he/she like to follow a strict routine? *If so*, what would happen if this was changed?

RED FLAGS

Developmental delay
No symbolic play by 2 years
No interactive play by 3 years
Lack of meaningful speech in short sentences by 3 years

SYSTEMS REVIEW (*SEE PAEDIATRIC HISTORY TEMPLATE*)

- **Development history** *(thorough)*
- **Pregnancy and birth history**
- **Immunisation history**
- **Feeding history** *(infants and toddlers)*

PATIENT'S PERSPECTIVE

- Feelings and effect on life – *already discussed*
- Ideas – Do you have any ideas yourself about what could be causing his/her behaviour?
- Concerns – Is there anything you are particularly concerned could be causing it? Is there anything in general that concerns you?
- Expectations – Was there anything in particular you were hoping for when you made the appointment for today?

BACKGROUND INFORMATION

PMH

- Does he/she suffer with any known behavioural conditions or learning difficulties?

DH

- Is he/she on any medications at the moment? Does he/she have any allergies?

FH

- Does anybody in the family have behaviour problems or learning difficulties?

SH

- How are things at home? Are there any problems? What are his/her siblings like?
- Has anyone at home ever been in trouble with the law?

CLOSING THE SESSION

- summary ± examination/explanation and planning/contract

DIFFERENTIAL DIAGNOSIS

ATTENTION DEFICIT HYPERACTIVITY DISORDER

- Usually affects children between the age of 3 and 7 years
- Inattention – Short attention span with difficulty concentrating in class
- Hyperactivity – Unable to sit still for long periods and constantly fidgeting
- Impulsiveness – Unable to wait in turn and little sense of danger
- Symptoms must be present for >6 months across at least two environments

CONDUCT DISORDER

- Usually affects children and adolescents above the age of 7 years
- Violence, bullying, theft, vandalism and cruelty to animals
- Problems at school, including truancy and often expulsion
- Disobedience and lack of respect for authority
- Can be precipitated by situation at home, including being bullied or abused, parental drug or alcohol addiction, family conflicts or big changes at home

AUTISTIC SPECTRUM DISORDER

- Social impairment – Lack of interest in playing with others/imaginary play
- Communication impairment – Delayed language development, few social gestures
- Repetitive behaviours – Deviating from set routines causes great difficulty to them; stereotypy is another feature (e.g. making particular sounds)
- Risk factors: gestational age <35 weeks, family history, chromosomal disorders, cerebral palsy

OTHER DIFFERENTIALS

- Oppositional defiant disorder – less severe variant of conduct disorder
- Hearing or visual impairment – evidence of developmental delay
- Learning difficulties
- Tic disorder e.g. Tourette's syndrome

INVESTIGATIONS

- Physical examination is required to rule out any medical causes
- Hearing assessment including audiometry if a concern is identified
- Speech and language assessment if developmentally delayed
- Multidisciplinary approach observing the child in different settings

MANAGEMENT

- A multidisciplinary approach is vital, involving the child, parents, paediatricians, general practitioners, psychologists, speech and language therapists, teachers, special education needs co-ordinators and others
- Autistic spectrum disorder – Behavioural modification, speech and language therapy, occupational therapy and the Treatment and Education of Autistic and Communication related handicapped CHildren (TEACCH) method are just some of many possible management strategies
- ADHD – Behavioural modification, parent education and family therapy; methylphenidate can be considered in moderate-to-severe cases of ADHD
- Conduct disorder – Behavioural modification and family therapy

FURTHER READING

NICE CKS on:
    ADHD, http://cks.nice.org.uk/attention-deficit-hyperactivity-disorder
    Conduct disorders, http://cks.nice.org.uk/conduct-disorders-in-children-and-young-people
    Autism, http://cks.nice.org.uk/autism-in-children

Psychiatry

LOW MOOD/DEPRESSION

INITIATING THE SESSION

- Greet the patient, ask an open question and screen for other problems

MEDICAL PERSPECTIVE

SEQUENCE OF EVENTS AND SYMPTOM ANALYSIS

- **Open question** – Can you tell me more about this?
- **Timeline** – How long have you felt like this? How did it all start? How have things progressed?
- **Ideas** – Can you think of any reason for feeling like this?
- **Effect on life** – How has this affected you?

CORE SYMPTOMS

- **Low mood** – How have you been feeling in yourself recently?
- **Anhedonia** – Are you able to get enjoyment from anything?
- **Fatigue** – How are your energy levels?

OTHER COMMON SYMPTOMS

- **Sleep** – Are you sleeping OK? Do you wake up earlier than you used to? How much earlier?
- **Appetite** – How is your appetite? Do you think you have lost any weight?
- **Libido** – How is your libido?

- **Diurnal variation** – Does your mood change at all during the day?
- **Concentration** – Are you able to concentrate when watching TV?
- **Self** – How do you feel about yourself right now? Do you have feelings of worthlessness or guilt?
- **Future/hopelessness** – How do you feel about the future?

RISK (*CONSIDER A MINI-SUMMARY JUST BEFORE THIS POINT*)

- It sounds like things have become very difficult for you lately; has it ever got so bad that you thought of harming yourself or others? *If yes, conduct full risk assessment, pp. 232*

SYSTEMS REVIEW

- **Bipolar** – Have you ever felt so good that other people said you were hyper and not yourself?
- **Psychosis** – Have you ever seen or heard things you couldn't quite explain?
- **Anxiety** – Do you ever feel particularly worried or anxious about anything?
- **Hypothyroidism** – You mentioned you have put on weight (*signposting*)…do you feel cold even when others say they are warm? *If yes, ask about other symptoms (e.g. menstrual abnormalities, dry puffy skin, hair thinning)*

PATIENT'S PERSPECTIVE

- **Feelings and effect on life** – *already covered*
- **Ideas** – *already covered*
- **Concerns** – Is there anything you are particularly concerned could be causing you to feel like this? Is there anything in general that concerns you?
- **Expectations** – Did you have anything in particular in mind you were hoping for when you made this appointment, or were you simply looking for some help?

BACKGROUND INFORMATION

PMH

- Have you ever suffered from any medical or psychiatric conditions? *If yes,* how long have you suffered from this for?
- *Ask about thyroid disease, depression, mania and schizophrenia*
- How would someone close to you have described you 2 years ago?

DH

- Are you taking any prescribed medications? Do you have any allergies?

FH

- Do any conditions run in your family?
- *Ask about depression and psychiatric illness generally*

SH

- Are you currently working? *If so,* what is your job? What does that involve?
- Can you tell me about your home situation (*occupants and any difficulties*)?
- Has your mood affected your job or home life in any way?
- Do you have family or friends to support you?
- Do you smoke? How many cigarettes do you smoke a day? How long for?
- Do you drink alcohol? How much do you drink in a week?
- Do you take any recreational drugs?

TO FINISH

- **Insight and support** – From what we have discussed, I feel you are suffering from depression. Do you agree? There is support and therapy available. Is this something you would be interested in talking about?
- **Follow-up** – I would like to see you again. Can we arrange a time to meet, perhaps next week? We could then discuss how to go forward from here.

CLOSING THE SESSION

- summary ± examination/explanation and planning/contract

IMPORTANT POINTS

- Be empathetic to the patients' concerns and how the symptoms have affected them. Good communication skills are particularly important in histories like this one
- Be sure to ask about past manic episodes and alcohol consumption as well as rule out organic causes such as hypothyroidism
- As with all psychiatric histories, never forget to properly assess risk
- There is less chance of further attempts in the immediate future if the patient has something to look forward to, so offer an early follow-up appointment

---

DIFFERENTIAL DIAGNOSIS

In a pressurised situation and with only a short time to take the history, practitioners may not remember to consider differential diagnoses for low mood. It is however very important not to fall into the trap of simply labelling the patient with depression without due consideration of the differentials. A few simple questions can ensure you have the correct diagnosis in mind. Dual diagnoses are common in psychiatry, so also consider the possibility of co-existing schizophrenia and anxiety. As well as those listed below, sleep-related disorders, dehydration and side effects of drugs such as beta-blockers can also cause low mood, whilst anaemia may primarily cause fatigue.

DEPRESSION

- Core symptoms – low mood, anhedonia and fatigue
- Typical symptoms – sleep disturbance, early morning waking (>2 h earlier than usual), decreased appetite, weight loss (>10%), decreased libido, diurnal mood variation,

feelings of worthlessness, guilt and hopelessness, decreased concentration and attention, recurrent thoughts of death/suicide
- Symptoms must be present for at least 2 weeks

BIPOLAR DISORDER

- Easy to miss diagnosis in OSCEs – Don't forget to ask about previous manic episodes
- Symptoms of mania include euphoria, grandiosity, flight of ideas, pressure of speech and a reduced need for sleep

SCHIZOAFFECTIVE DISORDER

- Ask about delusions and hallucinations

HYPOTHYROIDISM

- If time, ask one simple screening question e.g. regarding intolerance of the cold
- Other symptoms include constipation, oligomenorrhoea and weight gain

INVESTIGATIONS

- Mental state examination
- Risk assessment
- Assess hydration status and perform thyroid exam
- FBC and TFTs

MANAGEMENT

MILD

- Regular exercise
- Advice on sleep hygiene (regular sleep times, appropriate environment)
- Psychosocial therapy – CBT

MODERATE TO SEVERE

- Regular exercise; advice on sleep hygiene; CBT
- Medication – SSRI
- High-intensity psychosocial intervention (CBT or interpersonal therapy)
- Immediate and considerable high risk to themselves or others
- Admit to psychiatric ward (use Mental Health Act if necessary)

FURTHER READING

NICE CKS on depression, http://cks.nice.org.uk/depression

ANXIETY

INITIATING THE SESSION

- Greet the patient, ask an open question and screen for other problems

MEDICAL PERSPECTIVE

SEQUENCE OF EVENTS AND SYMPTOM ANALYSIS

- **Open question** – Can you tell me a bit more about what has been happening?
- **Timeline** – How long have you felt like this? How did it all start? How have things progressed?
- **Description** – Can you describe to me exactly what it is like/what happens when these worries come on?
- **Ideas** – Can you think of any reason for feeling like this?
- **Effect on life** – How has this affected you?

SYSTEMS REVIEW

- **Autonomic symptoms** – Have you noticed a dry mouth when the anxiety comes on? Sweating? Tremor? Sickly feeling? Awareness of your heart beating quickly? Pain anywhere?
- **Panic attack** – Are you ever overcome by sudden feelings of panic that seem to hit you out of the blue? What happens exactly? How long does it last?
- **Specific phobia versus generalised anxiety** – Is there a particular time, place or situation where these feelings come on or does it come on any time? Do you feel on edge all the time? Would you describe yourself as a worrier?
- **Obsessive compulsive disorder** – Do you get repetitive intrusive thoughts which you cannot resist? *If so*, what happens when you get these thoughts? Do you have any rituals or routines that you feel compelled to follow? *If so*, how would you feel if you did not follow them?
- **Depression with secondary anxiety** – Do you ever feel low in mood? Do you think you could be depressed?
- **Hyperthyroidism** – Have you noticed any change in your weight or appetite? Any change in the regularity or intensity of your periods?

> **RED FLAGS**
> *Chest pain – rule out ACS!*
> *Dual diagnoses e.g. depression*
> *Thoughts of DSH/suicide attempts*
> *Severe symptoms affecting function*

RISK

- I'm sorry but it is important that I ask this; have you ever had any thoughts of harming yourself?

PATIENT'S PERSPECTIVE

- **Feelings and effect on life** – *already covered*
- **Ideas** – *already covered*
- **Concerns** – Is there anything you are particularly concerned could be causing you to feel like this? Is there anything in general that concerns you?
- **Expectations** – Did you have anything in particular in mind you were hoping for when you made this appointment, or were you simply looking for some help?

BACKGROUND INFORMATION

PMH

- How would someone close to you have described you a few years ago? If relevant, have you always been a worrier?
- Do you suffer from any medical or psychiatric conditions?

DH

- Are you currently taking any medication? Are you allergic to any medications?
- How would you feel about taking medication to help if it was appropriate?

FH

- Do any conditions run in your family?
- Has anyone else in your family suffered from similar problems?

SH

- Are you currently working? *If so,* what is your job? What does that involve?
- Can you tell me about your home situation (*occupants and any difficulties*)?
- Have your anxieties affected your job or home life in any way?
- Do you have family or friends to support you?
- Do you smoke? How many cigarettes do you smoke a day? How long for?
- Do you drink alcohol? How much do you drink in a week?
- Do you use any recreational drugs?

CLOSING THE SESSION

- summary ± examination/explanation and planning/contract

IMPORTANT POINTS

- Must rule out organic causes – always consider if it could be cardiac in origin
- In histories such as this your communication skills are vitally important to obtaining a good mark – Build rapport with the patient and start the history empathetically e.g. "I can see you're upset, it must have been difficult for you to come here today." How has this affected their life? Some patients simply cannot function at all with anxiety and even seeing the doctor could be traumatic
- It is difficult/impossible to do a full history for anxiety in less than 10 minutes, but if you have time, asking about their childhood may reveal events that could have influenced their present state

DIFFERENTIAL DIAGNOSIS

The most important aspect of this history is to make sure the symptoms don't have an organic cause. If in any doubt, spend more time asking them questions regarding the cardiorespiratory systems in particular. If you spend all your time asking anxiety-related questions and the patient actually has an arrhythmia then your chances of passing this particular station will not be high!

GENERAL SYMPTOMS OF AN ANXIETY DISORDER

- Autonomic arousal – Palpitations, sweating, tremor, dry mouth
- Chest and abdominal symptoms – Breathing difficulty, feeling of choking, chest pain, nausea or abdominal distress (e.g. churning in stomach)
- Symptoms involving mental state – Feeling dizzy or fearful
- General symptoms – Hot flushes, cold chills, numbness, restlessness, feeling tense or irritable

GENERALISED ANXIETY DISORDER

- Feeling tense and worried by everyday situations
- Symptoms must have been present for at least 6 months
- The anxiety cannot be due to a physical disorder such as hyperthyroidism

PANIC ATTACK

- Unpredictable recurrent episodes of severe anxiety
- Sudden onset and lasts a few minutes
- Not associated with marked exertion or exposure to dangerous situations

PHOBIC ANXIETY DISORDERS (AGORAPHOBIA, SOCIAL AND SPECIFIC PHOBIAS)

- Anxiety evoked by particular situations leading to significant emotional distress
- Subsequent avoidance of these particular situations
- Includes a panic attack which occurs in an established phobic situation
- Agoraphobia includes fears of leaving home, public places, crowds, travelling alone
- Social phobia is a fear of scrutiny by others and consequently social situations
- Specific phobias are phobias restricted to highly specific situations (e.g. heights or flying)

ACUTE STRESS REACTION

- Develops quickly after an unexpected life crisis
- Symptoms settle within hours–days

POST-TRAUMATIC STRESS DISORDER

- Develops weeks–months after the trauma of a threatening or catastrophic event (e.g. a life-threatening situation or sexual abuse)
- Typical features include flashbacks, nightmares, detachment, anxiety, depression and avoiding anything that may trigger memories of the trauma

CARDIOGENIC CAUSES

- Angina/ACS – Crushing central chest pain radiating to arm/jaw on exertion
- Atrial fibrillation – Palpitations and shortness of breath (typical anxiety symptoms unlikely)

HYPERTHYROIDISM

- Non-specific symptoms include anxiety, tremor, sweating, palpitations, irritability
- Weight loss despite increased appetite, oligomenorrhoea, diarrhoea, ophthalmopathy and a goitre all indicate a diagnosis of hyperthyroidism

ALCOHOL WITHDRAWAL

- Causes non-specific symptoms of anxiety, nausea, sweating, tremor and irritability
- In severe form, delirium tremens, hallucinations, fever and seizures may occur
- History of alcohol abuse is imperative to making diagnosis

HYPOGLYCAEMIA

- Most commonly seen in diabetes with mistakes in timing or amount of insulin taken

INVESTIGATIONS

- Physical examination to look for signs of hyperthyroidism and cardiac disease
- Bloods – TFTs and glucose
- Blood pressure (phaeochromocytoma – rare)

MANAGEMENT

- Counselling
- Psychotherapy – CBT
- Relaxation training
- Medication – Beta-blockers and SSRIs

FURTHER READING

NICE CKS on generalised anxiety disorder, http://cks.nice.org.uk/generalized-anxiety-disorder

HALLUCINATIONS/DELUSIONS

INITIATING THE SESSION

- Greet the patient, ask an open question and screen for other problems

MEDICAL PERSPECTIVE

SEQUENCE OF EVENTS AND SYMPTOM ANALYSIS

- **Open question** – Can you tell me a bit more about what has been happening?
- **Exploration** – I understand you have been under a lot of stress recently. Sometimes when people are under stress they can have strange or unusual experiences, such as hearing voices, seeing strange things or feeling paranoid. Have you had any of these experiences yourself? What have you noticed?
- **Timeline** – How long have you felt like this? How did it all start? How have things progressed?

AUDITORY HALLUCINATIONS

- **Open question** – Can you tell me about the voices? How many are there?
- **True/false** – Where do you hear them – inside or outside your head? Can you ever stop them?
- **Second/third person** – Do they talk to you or about you?
- **Commands** – Do they ask you to do things? *If so,* what do they ask you to do?
- **Running commentary** – Do you hear them like a running commentary?

RED FLAGS

Loss of functioning
Risk to self or others
Command hallucinations
Grandiose delusions

OTHER HALLUCINATIONS (VISUAL, GUSTATORY, OLFACTORY)

- **Visual** – Do you see things that others can't? *If so,* can you describe them to me? When did you first notice this? How have things progressed since?
- **Gustatory/olfactory** – Have you noticed any strange tastes or smells that you couldn't explain? When did this start? How have things progressed?

DELUSIONS

- **Persecutory** – Do you feel anyone is out to get you?
- **Reference** – Does the newspaper, radio or television refer about you?
- **Control** – Is anyone trying to control you?
- **Passivity** – Is anyone trying to control your actions or feelings?
- **Grandiose** – Do you feel you have any special powers or abilities?
- **Nihilistic** – Do you feel your organs are rotting?

Whatever the type of delusion, ask about how long it has been going on for and check the fixity by gently challenging it (e.g. how sure are you about that?).

RULING OUT OTHER PSYCHIATRIC DIAGNOSES

- How has your mood been? Have you ever been diagnosed with depression, mania or anxiety?

RISK ASSESSMENT

- I can see you have clearly been under a lot of stress recently, have things ever got so bad that you've thought of harming yourself at all? Have things ever reached a stage where you have thought of harming others?

PATIENT'S PERSPECTIVE

- **Feelings and effect on life** – What effect has all of this had on your day-to-day life?
- **Ideas** – Do you have any ideas why you feel the way you do at the moment?
- **Concerns** – Is there anything you are particularly concerned could be causing you to feel like this? Is there anything in general that concerns you?
- **Expectations** – Did you have anything in particular in mind you were hoping for when you made this appointment, or were you simply looking for some help?

BACKGROUND INFORMATION

PMH

- Have you ever suffered from any medical or psychiatric conditions?

DH

- Are you currently taking any medications? Do you have any allergies?

FH

- Do any medical or psychiatric conditions run in your family?

SH

- Are you currently working? *If so,* what is your job? What does that involve?
- Can you tell me about your home situation (*occupants and any difficulties*)?
- Has your problem affected your job or home life in any way?
- Do you drink alcohol? Do you smoke? How much?
- Who is at home with you? Do you have much support from friends and family?

TO FINISH

- **Insight** – If I were to say as a doctor I thought you had a psychiatric problem, how would you feel about that? Would you take treatment for this if a psychiatrist felt it was appropriate?

CLOSING THE SESSION

- summary ± examination/explanation and planning/contract

- This history may present with another complaint (e.g. headache) in which you notice the patient is acting strangely (they may have seemingly delusional thoughts; appear dishevelled and agitated; or even respond to their hallucinations during the consultation)
- It may also present with a patient being brought in by the police or by friends and/or family due to concerns about their behaviour
- Offer plenty of reassurance and empathy before firing closed questions
- Try to connect with your patient's symptoms
- If presenting with a headache or other complaint, then be sure to ask relevant questions about that complaint first as even psychiatric patients can get ill!

DIFFERENTIAL DIAGNOSIS

SCHIZOPHRENIA

- Schneider's first-rank symptoms – Auditory hallucinations, delusions of perception, delusions of control and thought echo, insertion, withdrawal and broadcasting
- Negative symptoms – Anhedonia, blunting of responses, poverty of speech and marked apathy
- Positive symptoms – Hallucinations of any modality, catatonia, neologisms and tangential speech
- Risk factors include family history, heavy cannabis use and social isolation
- High risk of suicide, so always assess risk!

DRUG-INDUCED PSYCHOSIS

- Many drugs, including alcohol, cannabis and LSD can either mimic psychosis through intoxication or cause a chronic hallucinosis in long-term misuse
- Withdrawal states such as delirium tremens can also mimic psychosis

DELIRIUM

- An acute confusional state common in the elderly
- Can be the mode of presentation for infection in the elderly (e.g. UTI)
- Other causes include drugs (e.g. morphine, steroids and benzodiazepines), alcohol abuse/ withdrawal, metabolic disturbances and stroke

DEPRESSION WITH PSYCHOSIS

- Core features of depression present (low mood, anhedonia and fatigue)
- Delusions are the most common psychotic symptoms in depression (e.g. delusions of guilt, paranoia, persecution and nihilism)
- Patient may believe they are being punished for previous wrongs or that they are responsible for acts which they clearly could not be responsible for
- Hallucinations may involve hearing voices that are heavily critical of them

MANIA

- Signs and symptoms include elated mood, high energy levels and self-esteem, grandiosity, flight of ideas and restlessness
- Delusions of grandiosity are often present, as may other delusions (e.g. persecutory) or even hallucinations
- Patient will be talking very fast, constantly switching between topics
- There may be a previous history of depression (bipolar disorder)

INVESTIGATIONS

- Full physical examination, including neurological examination
- Mental state examination
- Bloods – FBC, U&Es, LFTs, TFTs, vitamin B12, blood glucose and folate
- Urine drug screen
- Chest x-ray
- If indicated – Serology for syphilis, lumbar puncture, EEG and MRI/CT brain

MANAGEMENT

- Biopsychosocial approach
- Psychological treatment – Psychotherapy and CBT
- Psychosocial rehabilitation – Psychoeducation; social worker (finances)
- Pharmacological treatment – Oral or intramuscular second generation (atypical) antipsychotic (e.g. risperidone or olanzapine)
- Treatment can be given in both outpatient or inpatient setting
- Inpatient setting indicated when patient is high risk to self or others – Use of the Mental Health Act may be necessary
- Community follow-up and close working with patient and family
- Electroconvulsive therapy can be used in catatonic schizophrenia

FURTHER READING

NICE CKS on psychosis, http://cks.nice.org.uk/psychosis-and-schizophrenia

FORGETFULNESS

INITIATING THE SESSION

- Greet the patient, ask an open question and screen for other problems

MEDICAL PERSPECTIVE

SEQUENCE OF EVENTS

- **Open question** – Can you tell me a bit more about what has been happening?
- **Timeline** – When did you first notice this? How have things progressed?

SYMPTOM ANALYSIS – COGNITION AND BEHAVIOUR

- **Short-term memory** – Do you have any difficulty remembering names? Appointments? Dates? Do you remember to take your medications every day?
- **Long-term memory** – Can you remember when you got married? What was your first job?
- **Visuospatial difficulties** – Do you have any difficulty recognising places, people or any items?
- **Language** – Do you ever struggle to find the right words when talking?
- **Behaviour** – Have you noticed any change in your behaviour? (*E.g. irritability, sexual disinhibition, wandering and social withdrawal.*)
- **Personality** – Have you noticed any changes in your personality? (*E.g. violence/outbursts, verbal/physical aggression.*)

SYSTEMS REVIEW

- **Depression** – How is your mood?
- **Anxiety** – Have you been feeling upset or anxious recently?
- **Psychosis** – I know this may sound silly, but have you seen or heard things that you couldn't quite explain?
- **Constitutional** – Have you been feeling unwell recently? Any fever?
- **Parkinsonism** – Have you noticed a tremor in either hand at all? Have you noticed any changes in your walking? Any changes in your handwriting?

RED FLAGS

Acute change in
cognition
Co-existent infection
Neurological symptoms
Loss of functioning
Lack of appropriate
support

RISK ASSESSMENT

- **Coping with activities of daily living** – Tell me about your current home situation. Are you coping? Are you able to wash yourself regularly? Dress yourself? Do the cleaning? Cooking? Shopping? How are things financially?
- **Dangerous events** – Have you had any falls? Have your neighbours or friends ever found you wandering the streets looking confused?
- **Driving** – Do you drive? *If so*, have you ever had any near-accidents? *If so*, what happened?
- **Harm** – I know things have been difficult recently, but have they ever got so bad that you've thought about harming yourself or others?

PATIENT'S PERSPECTIVE

- **Feelings and effect on life** – What effect has all of this had on your day-to-day life?
- **Ideas** – Why do you think you have been more forgetful recently?
- **Concerns** – Some people with this problem are concerned they may have dementia. Is this something you are worried about? Is there anything else you are concerned about?
- **Expectations** – Did you have anything in particular in mind you were hoping for when you made this appointment?

BACKGROUND INFORMATION

PMH

- Do you suffer from any medical or psychiatric conditions?
- *Ask specifically about hearing problems and visual difficulties*

DH

- Are you currently taking any medications? Do you remember to take them every day?
- Do you have any allergies?

FH

- Do any conditions run in your family?
- *Ask specifically about dementia*

SH

- Are you still working? *If working,* what do you do? How has this affected your job?
- Can you tell me about your home situation (*occupants and any difficulties*)?
- Do you have a husband/wife? Children? Grandchildren? Are your family able to offer much support?
- Has your memory affected your job or home life in any way?
- Do you smoke? Do you drink alcohol? How much?

TO FINISH

- **Collateral history** – Thank you for talking to me, I would like to talk to one of your close family or friends who have been concerned about you to ask them some questions. Is that OK with you?

CLOSING THE SESSION

- summary ± examination/explanation and planning/contract

DIFFERENTIAL DIAGNOSIS

ALZHEIMER'S DISEASE

- Progressive global impairment of cognitive functioning
- Short-term memory often affected first, followed by confusion, irritability, aggression, long-term memory loss, mood swings and incontinence
- Most common form of dementia, accounting for over half of the cases
- Risk factors include advanced age, Caucasian race, female sex and vascular disease

VASCULAR DEMENTIA

- Stepwise decline in cognitive functioning over months–years
- Evidence of previous stroke with onset of dementia within 3 months of stroke
- Cardiovascular risk factor likely to be present

DEMENTIA WITH LEWY BODIES

- Fluctuating confusion
- Parkinsonian features (e.g. tremor, bradykinesia, festinating gait and ataxia leading to falls and micrographia), visual hallucinations and intermittent loss of consciousness
- Short-term memory often preserved to a greater extent than in Alzheimer's, but visuospatial difficulties are more pronounced

FRONTO-TEMPORAL DEMENTIA

- Aggression, inappropriate social behaviour, emotional blunting, incontinence and speech and language difficulties all tend to occur early
- Often insidious with an earlier age of onset than in Alzheimer's disease

OTHER CAUSES (INCLUDING ORGANIC)

- Normal ageing process – Impairment of memory and intellect are common in the elderly but does not always justify a diagnosis of dementia!
- Delirium – Acute confusional state common in the elderly, often due to infection, drugs (e.g. morphine) or alcohol
- Depressive pseudodementia – Common in the elderly; often present with memory impairment and difficulty in attention and concentration
- Metabolic disturbances – E.g. uraemia from renal or liver failure, hypothyroidism, hypo-/hyper-calcaemia, hypoglycaemia and vitamin B12 deficiency

- Brain tumour – Behavioural/personality changes, headaches, seizures and nausea and vomiting are common features; usually a secondary tumour
- Parkinson's disease – Parkinsonian features preceding symptoms of dementia by at least 1 year

INVESTIGATIONS

Note: It is of paramount importance in dementia to rule out organic causes

- Full physical examination, including thyroid status
- Mini-mental state examination
- Bloods – FBC, U&Es, LFTs, TFTs, vitamin B12, blood glucose and folate
- Blood cultures
- Chest x-ray
- EEG
- MRI/CT brain
- Lumbar puncture (if Creutzfeldt–Jakob disease suspected)
- If needed – Serology for syphilis, PET scan and DAT Scan

MANAGEMENT

- Treat the underlying cause (if treatable) – E.g. Management of thyroid disease, B12 deficiency, shunting in hydrocephalus, levodopa in Parkinson's etc.
- Symptomatic – Environmental manipulation; lifestyle factors e.g. exercise, reduce alcohol and smoking, and encourage reading
- Supportive care for the family (including social worker input) – Caring for people with dementia is very demanding and can place a lot of stress on families; it is also important to consider the health and wellbeing of the carer
- Alzheimer's disease – Memory enhancing drugs e.g. rivastigmine
- Advice from DVLA after diagnosis of dementia
- Late stages of dementia – Residential or nursing homes may be the last option

FURTHER READING

NICE CKS on dementia, http://cks.nice.org.uk/dementia

MANIA

"I feel on top of the world doctor!"

"My partner has been upset for some reason and dragged me here, but I feel great doctor and have so many things to do..."

INITIATING THE SESSION

- Greet the patient, ask an open question and screen for other problems

MEDICAL PERSPECTIVE

SEQUENCE OF EVENTS

- **Open question** – Can you tell me a bit more about what has been happening?
- **Clarify** – Can I just check what you mean/what your partner was worried about?
- **Timeline** – When did you first notice this? How have things progressed? How have things been recently?

SYMPTOM ANALYSIS – KEY FEATURES

- **Reflect** – *Reflect on the manic features as you notice them (spell it out for your examiner!)*
- **Elated mood** – How are you feeling in yourself? How is your mood on a scale of 1–10? *Patient most likely will have already volunteered this information!*
- **High energy levels** – How are your energy levels?
- **High self-esteem** – How would you describe your self-esteem?
- **Grandiosity** – Do you have any special powers or abilities? Can you communicate with god? Do you think you can fly? *If yes, risk assess!*
- **Flight of ideas** (*Reflect back to the patient if he/she is very talkative and switching topics mid-conversation without letting you get a word in!*)

> **RED FLAGS**
>
> Loss of functioning
> Risk to self or others
> Grandiose delusions
> Trouble with police

BIOLOGICAL SYMPTOMS

- **Restlessness** – How is your sleep? (*I don't have time to sleep*)
- **Poor appetite** – How is your appetite? (*I eat when I feel hungry, but I don't have time to eat*)
- **Increased libido** – How is your sex drive? Do you have a regular partner? Have you slept with anyone else recently? Have you ever paid for sex?

RISK ASSESSMENT

- **Overspending** – Do you ever go on shopping binges? How are things financially?
- **Police** – Have you got into any trouble with the police recently? *If so*, why?
- **Self-harm/suicide** – Have you ever tried to harm yourself? *If present*, have you ever tried to use your special power(s)? *If so*, what happened?

SYSTEMS REVIEW – RULING OUT OTHER DIAGNOSES

- **Bipolar** – I know you feel great now, but have you ever been depressed?
- **Anxiety** – Do you ever feel particularly worried or anxious about anything?
- **Psychosis** – Have you ever seen or heard things that you couldn't quite explain?

PATIENT'S PERSPECTIVE

- **Feelings and effect on life** – What effect has all of this had on your day-to-day life?
- **Ideas** – Do you have any ideas about why you feel the way you do at the moment?
- **Concerns** – Is there anything you are particularly concerned could be causing you to feel like this? Is there anything in general that concerns you?
- **Expectations** – When you made the appointment for today, did you have anything in mind that you were hoping for?

BACKGROUND INFORMATION

PMH

- Have you ever been diagnosed with any medical or psychiatric conditions?
- *Ask about thyroid disease*

DH

- Do you take any medications? Do you have any allergies?

FH

- Do any conditions run in your family?

SH

- Are you currently working? *If so,* what is your job? What does that involve?
- Can you tell me about your home situation (*occupants and any difficulties*)?
- Have your family and friends been upset by any of your behaviour recently? *If so,* can you tell me why? How does your partner feel about what's been happening?
- Has your problem affected your job or home life in any way?
- Do you drink alcohol? How much do you drink in a week? Do you binge-drink?
- Do you use any recreational drugs? *If so,* when did you start? What do you use?
- Do you smoke? How many do you smoke in a week? For how many years?

CLOSING THE SESSION

- summary ± examination/explanation and planning/contract

IMPORTANT POINTS

- A manic patient might be very talkative during the interview. It is best not to interrupt them in the first 1–2 minutes, but it may be necessary after this due to time constraints e.g. "I'm sorry to interrupt you but can I please ask…"

- Alternatively, in a difficult scenario the patient may have some control over his/her symptoms and try to appear normal after being forced to come by his/her family/friends – Here, taking a collateral history is particularly important
- The best way to show to the examiner that you can elicit the mania history is to reflect back to the patient:
  - If the patient is talking rapidly – "You seem to talk quite fast" (pressured speech)
  - If the patient is saying lots of things, jumping from topic to topic – "You seem to have lots of ideas" (flight of ideas)
  - If the patient says I can talk to god – "You seem to have special powers"

DIFFERENTIAL DIAGNOSIS

MANIA

- Signs and symptoms include elated mood, high energy levels and self-esteem, grandiosity, flight of ideas and restlessness
- Patient will be talking very fast, constantly switching between topics
- Patient engages in pleasurable activities without considering negative consequences (e.g. sexual disinhibition, whilst not considering contraception)
- Shopping sprees are often described with money the patient does not have, therefore creating large amounts of debt and sometimes involving the police
- Delusions of grandiosity are often present, as may other delusions (e.g. persecutory) or even hallucinations
- Can have profound effect upon relationships with friends and family

HYPOMANIA

- Persistent, milder form of mania, with slightly elevated mood that alternates with irritability, high energy levels and restlessness
- Delusions and hallucinations are not present

BIPOLAR AFFECTIVE DISORDER

- Manic symptoms in a patient with a previous history of depression

SCHIZOAFFECTIVE DISORDER

- Significant history of manic and/or depressive episodes concurrent with symptoms of schizophrenia
- Schneider's first-rank symptoms – Auditory hallucinations, delusions of perception, delusions of control and thought echo, insertion, withdrawal and broadcasting
- Risk factors include family history, heavy cannabis use and social isolation

DRUG-INDUCED PSYCHOSIS

- Many drugs, including alcohol, cannabis and LSD, can either mimic psychosis through intoxication or cause a chronic hallucinosis in long-term misuse
- Withdrawal states such as delirium tremens can also mimic psychosis

ADJUSTMENT DISORDER

- Insomnia, poor concentration, avoiding important jobs, skipping school/work are signs that may mimic mania
- Low mood and anxiety in the context of an identifiable stressor help distinguish the disorder from other diagnoses

INVESTIGATIONS

- Physical examination, including assessment for a goitre
- Mental state examination
- Bloods – FBC, U&Es, LFTs, TFTs, vitamin B12, blood glucose and folate
- Urine drug screen
- Chest x-ray
- If indicated – Lumbar puncture and MRI/CT brain

MANAGEMENT

- Biopsychosocial approach
- Psychological – CBT, interpersonal therapy and family therapy
- Psychoeducation and vocational rehabilitation
- Pharmacological – Mood stabilisers (e.g. lithium); antipsychotics (e.g. olanzapine); benzodiazepines (e.g. lorazepam) to help insomnia/restlessness; antidepressants only used in selected cases as they can induce a manic episode
- Treatment can be given in both outpatient or inpatient setting
- Inpatient setting indicated when patient is high risk to self or others

FURTHER READING

NICE CKS on bipolar disorder, http://cks.nice.org.uk/bipolar-disorder

ALCOHOL HISTORY

"My wife thinks I have a problem with alcohol and made me see you today."
  "I think I'm developing a problem with alcohol."

INITIATING THE SESSION

- Greet the patient, ask an open question and screen for other problems

MEDICAL PERSPECTIVE

Sequence of events and symptom analysis

- **Open question** – Can you tell me about your drinking?
- **Timeline** – When did you first notice this? How have things progressed? What are things like now?
- **Drinking routine** – Starting from first thing in the morning, talk me through what you drink in a typical day (*what, how much, when and where?*)

  AUDIT questionnaire[1] – *See* Table 12.1.
  This is a screening test and is helpful to determine both whether there is a problem with alcohol and how severe the problem is, particularly if the patient does not have insight into their drinking problem. It can help aid further management.

FEATURES OF DEPENDENCE

- **Compulsion** – Do you get any cravings or urges for alcohol?
- **Control** – Do you have difficulty controlling your drinking once you start?
- **Withdrawal** –What happens when you don't drink? Do you get shakes or sweats when you don't drink for few days?
- **Tolerance** – Do you have to drink more to get the same effect you used to?
- **Primacy** – Would you say drinking has become your main priority in life?

IMPACT ON LIFE

- Has your drinking caused any problems in your life?
- **Work** – How has your drinking affected your working life? How are things financially for you currently?
- **Relationships** – Who is at home with you? How has your drinking affected your relationships with friends and family?
- **Law** – Have you had any problems with the law? Do you ever drive after drinking?

COMPLICATIONS

- **Physical complications** – Have you noticed any weight loss? How is your appetite? What is your diet like? Have you had any problems with your memory?
- **Depression/anxiety** – How has your mood been over the past few weeks?

RED FLAGS

Features of dependence
Co-existent psychiatric disorder
Significant impact on life
Physical complications

Table 12.1 The AUDIT questionnaire

Questions	0 points	1 point	2 points	3 points	4 points
Q1: How often do you have a drink that contains alcohol?	Never	Monthly or less	2–4 times a month	2–3 times a week	4+ times a week
Q2: How many standard alcoholic drinks do you have on a typical day when you are drinking?	1–2	3–4	5–6	7–9	10+
Q3: How often do you have 6 or more standard drinks on one occasion? *Skip to Q9+10 if total score for Q2+3 = 0*	Never	Less than monthly	Monthly	Weekly	Daily or almost daily
Q4: How often in the last year have you found you were not able to stop drinking once you had started?	Never	Less than monthly	Monthly	Weekly	Daily or almost daily
Q5: How often in the last year have you failed to do what was expected of you because of drinking?	Never	Less than monthly	Monthly	Weekly	Daily or almost daily
Q6: How often in the last year have you needed an alcoholic drink in the morning to get you going?	Never	Less than monthly	Monthly	Weekly	Daily or almost daily
Q7: How often in the last year have you had a feeling of guilt or regret after drinking?	Never	Less than monthly	Monthly	Weekly	Daily or almost daily
Q8: How often in the last year have you not been able to remember what happened when drinking the night before?	Never	Less than monthly	Monthly	Weekly	Daily or almost daily
Q9: Have you or someone else been injured as a result of your drinking?	No		Yes, but not last year		Yes, during the last year
Q10: Has a relative/friend/doctor/health worker been concerned about your drinking or advised you to cut down?	No		Yes, but not last year		Yes, during the last year
Score	1–7	8–15	16–19	20+	
Risk	Low risk	Hazardous drinking	Harmful drinking	Possible alcohol dependence	

Source: Reproduced from Babor et al. 2001. The Alcohol Use Disorders Identification Test: Guidelines for Use in Primary Care, 2nd ed. World Health Organization. With permission.

- **Psychosis** – Have you noticed any strange or unusual experiences?
- **Self-harm/suicide** – It seems as if things have been very difficult for you recently, have things ever got so bad that you thought about harming yourself?

PATIENT'S PERSPECTIVE

- **Feelings and effect on life** – What effect has your drinking had on day-to-day life?
- **Ideas** – How do you feel about your drinking? Do you think it is a problem?

- **Concerns** – Is there anything you are concerned about?
- **Expectations** – When you made the appointment for today, did you have anything in mind that you were hoping for?

BACKGROUND INFORMATION

PMH

- Do you suffer from any medical or psychiatric conditions?
- Have you ever had any treatments or detox for alcohol? What helped? What triggered your relapse?

DH

- Are you currently taking any medications? Do you have any allergies?

FH

- Has anyone in your family had problems with alcohol?
- Do any conditions run in your family?

SH

- Are you currently working? *If so,* what is your job? What does that involve?
- Can you tell me about your home situation (*occupants and any difficulties*)?
- Has alcohol affected your job or home life in any way?
- Do you smoke?
- Do you use any recreational drugs?

INSIGHT

It seems alcohol has been a significant part of your life...

- Do you think you have a drink problem?
- Do you want to stop or reduce your drinking?
- Would you be interested in accepting help if offered to you?

CLOSING THE SESSION

- summary ± examination/explanation and planning/contract

IMPORTANT POINTS

- It is important to develop a rapport with the patient before asking personal questions about their drinking habits; otherwise patients are likely to be resistive and potentially dishonest to your questioning
- It is important to take a holistic approach to an alcohol history. It is important to know what effect alcohol has had on their life, just as it is important to find any potential complications arising from alcohol abuse

- Never forget to assess risk in a psychiatric history
- A similar approach can be used when taking a recreational drugs history
- The AUDIT questionnaire is very useful in primary and secondary care. In the time-limited nature of the OSCEs, however, it may be more important to ascertain their drinking routine, the impact it has had on their life and any symptoms of complications. If the patient already accepts they have a problem with alcohol, then it may be enough to mention at the end of your OSCE you would also do the AUDIT questionnaire if you had more time

DIFFERENTIAL DIAGNOSIS

Alcoholism is suggested by all the features mentioned in this history. Differentials for this history are not relevant as the key aspect is to see whether the candidate can ascertain all the important information about the patient's drinking.

INVESTIGATIONS

- General physical examination, involving assessing for malnourishment, signs of liver disease and signs of heart disease (including atrial fibrillation and alcoholic cardiomyopathy)
- Bloods to screen for secondary damage – FBC (macrocytic anaemia), U&Es, CRP, LFTs, clotting screen, lipids, glucose, gamma-GT and vitamin levels (particularly thiamine)
- Further investigations depend on any related illness e.g. abdominal ultrasound and CT/MRI abdomen (for liver disease) and echocardiography (for heart disease)

MANAGEMENT

GENERAL MEASURES

- Advice about the adverse effects of alcohol
- Vitamin supplements, including thiamine to prevent Wernicke's encephalopathy and vitamin B co-strong
- Support and advice (including a listening ear at times)
- Financial support (you can signpost to the Citizens Advice Bureau)

ACUTE ALCOHOL WITHDRAWAL

- Consider whether the patient needs inpatient management
- IV Pabrinex or oral thiamine to prevent Wernicke's encephalopathy
- Chordiazepoxide to treat tremor and agitation in delirium tremens

ABSTINENCE

- Social support – Involve family and friends in their care where possible
- Support groups, including Alcoholics Anonymous or similar groups
- CBT
- Acamprosate – Reduces cravings
- Naltrexone – Reduces pleasurable effects of alcohol; particularly effective in binge drinkers
- Disulfiram – Causes an unpleasant reaction if the patient drinks alcohol, including nausea, headache and palpitations

REFERENCE

1. The AUDIT questionnaire. Babor TF, Higgins-Biddle JC, Saunders JB and Monteiro MG (2001). The Alcohol Use Disorders Identification Test: Guidelines for Use in Primary Care, 2nd ed. World Health Organization.

FURTHER READING

NICE CKS on alcoholism, http://cks.nice.org.uk/alcohol-problem-drinking

EATING DISORDER

"I don't know why I've been dragged here, everything is fine…"
"Mum brought me in because she thinks I'm not eating…"
"I was wondering if there was anything you could do to help me lose some weight?"

INITIATING THE SESSION

- Greet the patient, ask an open question and screen for other problems

MEDICAL PERSPECTIVE

SEQUENCE OF EVENTS

- **Open questions** – What do you think makes your *mum/dad/friend* worry about your eating? Can you tell me a bit more about your eating?
- **Timeline** – When do you think this all started? How has it progressed since then?
- **Ideas** – Can you think of any reason you have/why your family thinks you have a problem with food? Do you think you have a problem with food? Do you worry about your weight?
- **Effect on life** – How do you feel in yourself? What effect has your eating had on your life?

At this point, it is important to show empathy to your patient and fully explore any cues given to develop rapport. Some of the questions that follow can feel intrusive to the patient unless you have developed a relationship first.

SYMPTOM ANALYSIS

- **Daily routine** – Can you describe what you eat in a typical day? *Start with first thing in the morning and clarify if the routine is fixed every day. Do they avoid eating with others*?
- **Fear of fatness** – How would you feel if you gained weight?
- **Weight** – Have you got a target weight you want to reach? I'm sorry, I know this is personal but can I ask how much you weigh? How tall are you? (*NB: Is there a BMI scale/ calculator in the room*?) Have you lost any weight?
- **Binging** – Do you ever binge on food? *If yes*, how do you feel afterwards? Do you do anything to counteract the binge? What do you do? Do you ever deliberately make yourself sick afterwards or use laxatives?
- **Maladaptive behaviours** – Have you ever made yourself throw up after eating? Do you exercise? How often? Have you ever used appetite suppressants or water tablets?

SCOFF QUESTIONNAIRE (*RECOGNISED SCREENING TOOL FOR EATING DISORDERS*)

- **Sick** – Do you make yourself *Sick* because you are uncomfortably full?
- **Control** – Do you worry that you have lost *Control* over how much you eat?
- **One stone** – Have you lost more than *One stone* (~6 kg) in the past 3 months?
- **Feel fat** – Do you believe you are *Fat* even when others think you are thin?
- **Food dominates** – Would you say that *Food* dominates your life?

SYSTEMS REVIEW

- Have you noticed any physical problems lately?
- **Amenorrhoea** – Have you been getting your periods regularly?
- **Quick screen** – How are your energy levels? Have you been feeling dizzy or faint? Have you noticed any change with your bowels? Have you noticed any changes to your hair? Do you get any chest pain or palpitations?
- **Risk** – From what you tell me I can see things have been difficult for you. Some people that go through similar things have thoughts of wanting to harm themselves in some way. Have you ever had thoughts like that?

PATIENT'S PERSPECTIVE

- **Feelings and effect on life** – *already covered*
- **Ideas** – *already covered*
- **Concerns** – Is there anything you are concerned about?
- **Expectations** – When you made the appointment for today, did you have anything in mind that you were hoping for?

BACKGROUND INFORMATION

PMH

- Do you suffer from any medical or psychiatric illnesses?
- *Ask specifically about diabetes*

DH

- Are you currently taking any medication?
- Are you taking anything to help lose weight such as laxatives, water tablets or appetite suppressants? *If so,* are you aware of the dangers these can pose?
- Do you have any allergies?

FH

- Do any conditions run in the family?
- *Ask about eating disorders and psychiatric disorders generally*

SH

- Are you currently working? *If so,* what is your job? What does that involve?
- Can you tell me about your home situation (*occupants and any difficulties*)?
- Has your problem affected your job or home life in any way?
- Have you had any difficulties in any relationships with friends, family or partners because of your weight? What do your friends think about your weight? Do they say anything? Are you in a relationship? What does he/she think?
- Do you smoke? Drink alcohol? How much?

CLOSING THE SESSION

- summary ± examination/explanation and planning/contract

DIFFERENTIAL DIAGNOSIS

It is very important to rule out possible organic causes if a patient is underweight. The key in eating disorders is that the patient has a distorted body image and wishes to lose weight. If they are concerned about their weight loss or their weight loss is unintended then careful questioning into possible organic causes is needed.

ANOREXIA NERVOSA

- Underweight (BMI <17.5 or a BMI below the 2.4th centile in those under 18 years)
- Distorted body image – think they are fat despite being told they are thin
- Fear of gaining weight
- Food dominates thinking – careful about what they eat; may lie when asked about food consumption
- May utilise other methods of weight loss such as excessive exercise (e.g. 2 hours every day), taking laxatives, diuretics or appetite suppressants
- Although more commonly a feature of bulimia, vomiting can also occur in anorexia
- Amenorrhoea/oligomenorrhoea are frequently present

BULIMIA NERVOSA

- Unlike in anorexia, likely to be of normal weight or overweight
- Binge eating – repetitive episodes of eating large amounts of food
- Compensatory behaviour – try to counteract the fattening effect of the binge by inducing vomiting (common), taking laxatives, diuretics, extreme dieting or exercise
- Binges and compensatory behaviour need to occur at least once a week for 3 months to meet diagnostic criteria
- Eating patterns are typically irregular
- Amenorrhoea/oligomenorrhoea may again occur
- Erosion of the teeth, continuous sore throat and reflux due to purging

BINGE EATING

- Recurrent binges of food with loss of control over quantity of food consumed
- Similar but different to bulimia in that no compensatory behaviour is observed

- Binges need to occur at least once a week for 3 months for diagnosis
- Weight may be normal or overweight (commonly occurs in obese individuals)

ATYPICAL EATING DISORDER/EATING DISORDER NOT OTHERWISE SPECIFIED

- Most common eating disorder seen in community
- Criteria for other eating disorders not met e.g. slightly above weight threshold for anorexia nervosa or binges not occurring frequently enough for bulimia nervosa

INVESTIGATIONS

- Further detailed history and mental state examination – psychiatric co-morbidities are common
- Blood pressure
- Assess for proximal myopathy
- Bloods – FBC, U&Es, glucose, LFTs, magnesium, bone profile
- ECG

MANAGEMENT

- Multidisciplinary approach required and usually co-ordinated in secondary care
- Consider admission if high risk, rapid weight loss, very low weight or signs of serious physical complications (eating disorders units are available throughout the UK)
- Dietary advice – nutrition, regular balanced meals etc. (consider dietician input)
- Psychotherapy – CBT or interpersonal therapy
- Medication – SSRIs (fluoxetine) can help reduce urge to binge and purge; or if co-morbid depression

FURTHER READING

NICE CKS on eating disorders, http://cks.nice.org.uk/eating-disorders

SELF-HARM/SUICIDE ATTEMPT (RISK ASSESSMENT)

INITIATING THE SESSION

- Greet the patient, ask an open question and screen for other problems

MEDICAL PERSPECTIVE

TO START

- How are you feeling today? I understand you took some tablets last night, I'm really sorry things got that bad for you

BEFORE

- **Prior events/mood** – If you don't mind me asking, what happened before that made you feel like you had to end it all/harm yourself? Have you been feeling low for a while?
- **Plan** – Did you plan to harm yourself? What plans did you make? How long had you been planning this for?
- **Precautions** – Did you try to make sure you wouldn't get caught, like locking the door or making sure you were alone?
- **Preparation** – Did you write a note or make a will in preparation?
- **Told anyone?** – Did you tell anybody about it before or seek help afterwards?

DURING

- **Sequence of events** – Can you talk me through exactly what happened? (*How*? *Where*? *When*?)
- **Expectations** – Did you expect to die?
- **Alcohol/drugs** – Were you under the influence of alcohol or drugs at the time?

AFTER

- **Discovery** – How were you discovered? Did you tell anyone?
- **Anger/regret** – How do you feel about what has happened?
- **Lingering thoughts** – Do you still have any thoughts of doing something like this again?

RED FLAGS

Violent method used
Planning in place
Ongoing suicidal intent
Attempt to avoid rescue
Previous suicide
   attempts
Access to a means of
   self-harm
Recent adverse life event

PATIENT'S PERSPECTIVE

- **Feelings and effect on life** – How has your mood affected your day-to-day life?
- **Ideas** – Why do you think you feel the way you do?
- **Concerns** – Is there anything you are particularly concerned about?
- **Expectations** – Is there anything in particular you feel you need help with?

BACKGROUND INFORMATION

PMH

- Do you suffer from any medical or psychiatric illnesses such as depression?
- Have you ever tried to take your life or harm yourself before this?

DH

- Are you currently taking any medication?
- Do you have stores of any medications at home?

FH

- Has anyone in your family ever tried to harm themself?

SH

- Are you currently working? What is your job? How are things at work?
- Who is at home? Do you have a partner or kids? Do you have friends around you?
- Do you drink alcohol? How much do you drink in a week?
- Do you take any recreational drugs?
- Do you think you need any help? Would you be prepared to accept any help?

TO FINISH

- **Follow-up** – I would like to see you again next week. Can we arrange a time to meet? Is there anything you would like to talk about?

CLOSING THE SESSION

- summary ± examination/explanation and planning/contract

IMPORTANT POINTS

- Empathise and establish rapport with patient before diving into what happened
- In the back of your mind consider if this patient is at risk of future attempts
- If intended suicide, did they plan and prepare the act to meet their intended outcome?
- Did they genuinely believe it would kill them or could it be a cry for attention? Pay careful attention to the method (e.g. Did they only take four paracetamol tablets?)
- There is less risk of the patient attempting self-harm in the immediate future if they have something to look forward to
- *Always* consider if there are any safeguarding issues e.g. you should notify social services if the patient has a dependent such as a young child they look after

DIFFERENTIAL DIAGNOSIS

SELF-HARM

- Deliberate act of self-harm with a non-fatal outcome done in the knowledge that it is potentially harmful
- Methods:
  - Overdose (NSAIDs most commonly; antidepressants)
  - Self-inflicted injuries (e.g. cutting self)

- Reasons for self-harm, the eight C's:
  - Coping mechanism
  - Control
  - Calming/comforting
  - Cleansing (e.g. from sexual abuse)
  - Confirmation of existence
  - Creating comfortable numbness
  - Chastisement (e.g. if depressed)
  - Communication
- Risk factors:
  - Age 16–24 years
  - Female
  - Recent stressful event
  - Personality disorder
  - Areas of high unemployment rate
- 10% lifetime suicide risk – risk highest in weeks following act

SUICIDE

- Deliberate act of self-harm with a fatal outcome done in the knowledge that the act is potentially fatal
- Methods:
  - Hanging
  - Self-poisoning (are they in a profession with access to dangerous chemicals?)
  - Drug/alcohol overdose
  - Gunshot (more common in USA)
- Risk factors:
  - Risk increases with age
  - Male
  - Lost job
  - Separated/divorced/widowed
  - Depression/mood disorder
  - Alcohol/drugs abuse
  - Serious physical illness
- Factors increasing likeliness of future suicide attempt:
  - Immediate intent after recent escalation
  - Well-constructed plan involving a violent method or with access to means
  - Likelihood of further bad news

INVESTIGATIONS

- Mental state examination
- Collaborative history from family/friend

MANAGEMENT

- Allow them to vent their emotions
- Identify possible coping mechanisms

- Bolster self-esteem
- Explore effects their suicide would have on family and friends
- Make plans for future
- Does this patient require inpatient admission?
- Ensure adequate support at home
- Give telephone number for mental health support with instructions if things get worse
- Remove access to means
- Regular planned follow-up

FURTHER READING

NICE CKS on self-harm, http://cks.nice.org.uk/self-harm

Index